MW00510477

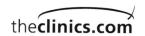
theclinics.com

CLINICS IN
SPORTS MEDICINE

Behind the Scenes
as a Team Physician

GUEST EDITOR
Jeff G. Konin, PhD, ATC, PT

CONSULTING EDITOR
Mark D. Miller, MD

April 2007 • Volume 26 • Number 2

SAUNDERS

An Imprint of Elsevier, Inc.
PHILADELPHIA   LONDON   TORONTO   MONTREAL   SYDNEY   TOKYO

W.B. SAUNDERS COMPANY
A Division of Elsevier Inc.

1600 John F. Kennedy Blvd. • Suite 1800 • Philadelphia, Pennsylvania 19103

http://www.theclinics.com

CLINICS IN SPORTS MEDICINE
April 2007
Editor: Debora Dellapena

Volume 26, Number 2
ISSN 0278-5919
ISBN-13: 978-1-4160-4297-6
ISBN-10: 1-4160-4297-0

Copyright © 2007 by Elsevier Inc. All rights reserved. No part of this publication may be reproduced or transmitted in any form or by any means, electronic or mechanical, including photocopy, recording, or any information retrieval system, without written permission from the Publisher.

Single photocopies of single articles may be made for personal use as allowed by national copyright laws. Permission of the publisher and payment of a fee is required for all other photocopying, including multiple or systematic copying, copying for advertising or promotional purposes, resale, and all forms of document delivery. Special rates are available for educational institutions that wish to make photocopies for non-profit educational classroom use. Permissions may be sought directly from Elsevier's Rights Department in Philadelphia, PA, USA: phone (+1) 215 239 3804, fax (+1) 215 239 3805, e-mail healthpermissions@elsevier.com. Requests may also be completed on-line via the Elsevier homepage (http://www.elsevier.com/locate/permissions). In the USA, users may clear permissions and make payments through the Copyright Clearance Center, Inc., 222 Rosewood Drive, Danvers, MA 01923, USA; phone: (978) 750-8400; fax: (978) 750-4744, and in the UK through the Copyright Licensing Agency Rapid Clearance Service (CLARCS), 90 Tottenham Court Road, London WIP 0LP, UK; phone (+44) 171 436 5931; fax: (+44) 171 436 3986. Other countries may have a local reprographic rights agency for payments.

Reprints: For copies of 100 or more, of articles in this publication, please contact the Commercial Reprints Department, Elsevier Inc., 360 Park Avenue South, New York, New York 10010-1710. Tel. (212) 633-3813; Fax: (212) 462-1935 e-mail: reprints@elsevier.com.

The ideas and opinions expressed in *Clinics in Sports Medicine* do not necessarily reflect those of the Publisher. The Publisher does not assume any responsibility for any injury and/or damage to persons or property arising out of or related to any use of the material contained in this periodical. The reader is advised to check the appropriate medical literature and the product information currently provided by the manufacturer of each drug to be administered to verify the dosage, the method and duration of administration, or contraindications. It is the responsibility of the treating physician or other health care professional, relying on independent experience and knowledge of the patient, to determine drug dosages and the best treatment for the patient. Mention of any product in this issue should not be construed as endorsement by the contributors, editors, or the Publisher of the product or manufacturers' claims.

Clinics in Sports Medicine (ISSN 0278-5919) is published quarterly by Elsevier Inc., 360 Park Avenue South, New York, NY 10010-1710. Months of publication are January, April, July, and October. Business and Editorial Offices: 1600 John F. Kennedy Blvd., Suite 1800, Philadelphia, PA 19103-2899. Customer Service Offices: 6277 Sea Harbor Drive, Orlando, FL 32887-4800. Periodicals postage paid at New York, NY, and additional mailing offices. Subscription prices are $205.00 per year (US individuals), $313.00 per year (US institutions), $103.00 per year (US students), $232.00 per year (Canadian individuals), $371.00 per year (Canadian institutions), $135.00 (Canadian students), $265.00 per year (foreign individuals), $371.00 per year (foreign institutions), and $135.00 per year (foreign students). Foreign air speed delivery is included in all *Clinics* subscription prices. All prices are subject to change without notice. POSTMASTER: Send address changes to *Clinics in Sports Medicine*, Elsevier Periodicals Customer Service, 6277 Sea Harbor Drive, Orlando, FL 32887-4800. **Customer Service: 1-800-654-2452 (US). From outside of the US, call 1-407-345-4000.** E-mail: hhspcs@harcourt.com.

Clinics in Sports Medicine is covered in *Index Medicus, Current Contents/Clinical Medicine, Excerpta Medica,* and *ISI/Biomed.*

Printed in the United States of America.

CLINICS IN SPORTS MEDICINE

Behind the Scenes as a Team Physician

SEVIER
UNDERS

CONSULTING EDITOR

MARK D. MILLER, MD, Professor, Department of Orthopaedic Surgery; Head, Division of Sports Medicine, University of Virginia Health System, Charlottesville, Virginia

GUEST EDITOR

JEFF G. KONIN, PhD, ATC, PT, Associate Professor, Department of Orthopaedic Surgery; Executive Director, Sports Medicine and Athletic Related Trauma (SMART) Institute College of Medicine, University of South Florida, Tampa, Florida

CONTRIBUTORS LIST

THOMAS E. ABDENOUR, MA ATC, Head Athletic Trainer, Golden State Warriors, Oakland, California

JON ALMQUIST, MS, ATC, Fairfax County Public Schools, Athletic Training Program, Falls Church, Virginia

JAMES R. ANDREWS, MD, Alabama Sports Medicine and Orthopaedic Center, Birmingham, Alabama

JOEL L. BOYD, MD, Associate Professor, University of Minnesota; Team Physician, Minnesota Wild, National Hockey League; Minnesota Vikings, National Football League; Minnesota Lynx, Women's Basketball League; Assistant Team Physician, Minnesota Timberwolves, National Basketball Association; TRIA Orthopedic Center, Bloomington, Minnesota

ANTHONY BUONCRISTIANI, MD, Fellow, Center for Sports Medicine, University of Pittsburgh Medical Center, Pittsburgh, Pennsylvania

JIM CLOVER, MEd, ATC, PTA, Instructor, Riverside County Office of Education Sports Therapy and Fitness; Owner, Clover Enterprises Inc., Riverside, California

PETER A. DOBROWOLSKI, BS, Divisions of Sports Medicine and Shoulder Surgery, Department of Orthopaedic Surgery, The Johns Hopkins University, Baltimore, Maryland

FREDDIE H. FU, MD, HDSc, David Silver Professor and Chairman, Department of Orthopaedic Surgery, University of Pittsburgh Medical Center, Pittsburgh, Pennsylvania

MIKE GOFORTH, MS, ATC, Director of Athletic Training, Eddie Ferrell Athletic Training Facility, Virginia Tech University, Blacksburg, Virginia

MARY LLOYD IRELAND, MD, Orthopaedic Surgeon and President, Kentucky Sports Medicine, Lexington, Kentucky

DAVID KNITTER, MD, Medical Director, Department of Sports Medicine; Team Physician, Center for Innovation in Health and Human Services, Department of Health Sciences, James Madison University, Harrisonburg, Virginia

JEFF G. KONIN, PhD, ATC, PT, Associate Professor, Department of Orthopaedic Surgery; Executive Director, Sports Medicine and Athletic Related Trauma (SMART) Institute, College of Medicine, University of South Florida, Tampa, Florida

TOM KUSTER, MS, ATC, NASM-PES, Assistant Director of Sports Medicine, Department of Sports Medicine, James Madison University, Harrisonburg, Virginia

JAMES KYLE, MD, Family, Athletic and Recreational Medicine, Ponte Vedra, Florida

JOE LEAMAN, MS, ATC, HEALTHSOUTH Sports Medicine and Rehabilitation Center, Vienna, West Virginia

LARRY LEMAK, MD, Interim Chair of Orthopaedics, University of South Florida; Chief Executive Officer, Sports Medicine and Athletic Related Trauma (SMART) Institute, University of South Florida Partner, Alabama Sports Medicine, Birmingham, Alabama; Medical Director, Major League Soccer; Medical Director, NFL Europa, Frankfurt, Germany

MARTIN MATNEY, MBA, MS, ATC, PTA, Clinic Manager, Whitesel ProTherapy, Inc., Kirkland, Washington

EDWARD G. MCFARLAND, MD, Divisions of Sports Medicine and Shoulder Surgery, Department of Orthopaedic Surgery, The Johns Hopkins University, Lutherville, Baltimore, Maryland

SCOTT MONTGOMERY, MD, Orthopedic Surgeon, Ochsner Sports Medicine, New Orleans, Louisiana

LENNY NAVITSKIS, MEd, ATC, CSCS, NREMT-I, Assistant Athletic Trainer, University of Georgia, Athens, Georgia

CHARLES COLE NOFSINGER, MD, MS, Assistant Professor and Team Physician, Department of Orthopaedic Surgery, University of South Florida, Tampa, Florida

MICHAEL PRYBICIEN, MA, ATC, CSCS, NREMT, Head Athletic Trainer, Passaic Board of Education, Passaic, New Jersey

J. SCOTT QUINBY, MD, Orthopedic Surgeon, Sports Medicine Clinic of North Texas; Baylor University Medical Center; Co-Director, Baylor Sports Advantage, Dallas, Texas

JOELLE STABILE REHBERG, DO, Montville Primary Care Physicians; Team Physician, Montville Township Public Schools, Montville, New Jersey

ROBB S. REHBERG, PhD, ATC, CSCS, NREMT, Assistant Professor and Coordinator of Athletic Training Clinical Education, Department of Exercise and Movement Sciences, William Paterson University, Wayne, New Jersey

UMASUTHAN SRIKUMARAN, MD, Divisions of Sports Medicine and Shoulder Surgery, Department of Orthopaedic Surgery, The Johns Hopkins University, Baltimore, Maryland

YOUXIN SU, MD, Divisions of Sports Medicine and Shoulder Surgery, Department of Orthopaedic Surgery, The Johns Hopkins University, Baltimore, Maryland

FOTIOS PAUL TJOUMAKARIS, MD, Fellow, Center for Sports Medicine, University of Pittsburgh Medical Center, Pittsburgh, Pennsylvania

JEROME WALL, MD, Director, The S.P.O.R.T. Clinic, Riverside, California

JAMES WHITESIDE, MD, American Sports Medicine Institute, Birmingham, Alabama

EVIER
NDERS

CLINICS IN SPORTS MEDICINE

Behind the Scenes as a Team Physician

CONTENTS VOLUME 26 • NUMBER 2 • APRIL 2007

> Being a team physician requires a whole new set of communications skills, depending on the organization one is affiliated with. There may be a single expected procedure to follow, or multiple procedures may be required. Regardless, it is imperative for the team physician to understand that his or her role is vital to those who seek accurate and timely information, thus potentially requiring physicians to adapt their current methods for communicating. Learning how to communicate as a team physician in a timely and accurate manner, understanding the appropriate chain of command, and avoiding common pitfalls associated with improper and sometimes adverse forms of communication will pave the way for an excellent long-term working relationship.

> The transition to the care of the college student-athlete carries with it a number of adjustments. In private practice it is customary to make medical decisions and initiate therapies from the confines of the examination room. The doctor-patient relationship is the principal focus. Although this relationship remains paramount in college athletics, the world of concerned and affected parties dramatically expands. It is in this context that the authors explore the concept of access in the role of a team physician. To use what is becoming an over used cliché, what makes one a valued team physician is being "the right person, in the right place at the right time."

> The team physician landscape is littered with political land mines. In the high-stakes world of professional sports, the politics of each encounter

and medical decision—from figuring out how to get hired, to setting up a communication chain of command, to treating visiting players, to fending off the media—must be identified, assessed, and resolved. Key information must be communicated according to the expectations and unique personalities of each owner, general manager, coach, trainer, and athlete. The best team physicians manage relationships, competing agendas, and politically charged circumstances as adeptly as they wield a scalpel.

Building a Sports Medicine Team 173

Freddie H. Fu, Fotios Paul Tjoumakaris, and
Anthony Buoncristiani

There have been a growing number of participants in high school and collegiate athletics in recent years, placing ever-increasing demands on the sports medicine team. Building a winning sports medicine team is equally as important to the success of an athletic organization as fielding talented athletes. Acquisition of highly qualified, motivated, and hardworking individuals is essential in providing high quality and efficient health care to the athlete. Maintaining open paths of communication between all members of the team is the biggest key to success and an optimal way to avoid confusion and pitfalls.

Establishing a New Practice as a Team Physician 181

J. Scott Quinby

The role of a team physician is an integral part of establishing a new practice. Regardless of the type of practice one enters, the team physician role provides an opportunity to establish an early referral base to build the foundation of a successful practice. Although this comes with great responsibility and significant time commitments, the joy of developing your practice doing what you enjoy most, sports medicine, makes these drawbacks less perceptible. Using all your potential resources and keeping your eye on the ball will simplify reaching the goal of having a happy, healthy, and rewarding career.

Balancing Life as a Team Physician 187

Mary Lloyd Ireland

This article reviews the author's ten commandments for a balanced life as a team physician: (1) Do the right thing, always, no exceptions; (2) It's better to be an advocate than curse your competition; (3) Don't demand respect from players and coaches, earn it; (4) Loyalty is the weakest of human values (5) Communicate: Team physicians must always be available to athletic training staff; (6) In order to hit the mark, one must aim a little higher; (7) Enjoy your role as team physician; (8) Remember the five A's—Availability, Ability, Affability, Advocacy, and Affiliation; (9) Dare to care; and (10) Don't forget your family and friends.

Team coverage can be the most rewarding and the most challenging aspect of a physician's career; however, evaluate the realistic risks and benefits of covering a team. Understand what the team is looking for. Prior physicians may have been dismissed for a specific action, may have left on their own, or may have been asked to pay for the privilege of serving. Tell the team what you have to offer and what you need to make the relationship work, and be prepared to walk away from the deal if the risks are too high. Understanding the implications of working without a contract and the elements of an appropriate contract is paramount to a successful relationship.

Athletes participate at many different levels of competition—from amateur to professional, from backyard sandlot to Yankee Stadium. There are as many different organized structures involved in providing medical care to athletes as there are types of athletes themselves. Although the organizational structures involved in providing medical care for a little league team in a small town are different from those involved in providing care for a professional baseball team, the mission is the same—caring for athletes. This is the central theme of this article. Though there are different organizational structures, there are more common threads than differences in the mission of those who provide medical care for athletes at any level.

Time is the greatest negative financial burden that you accept as a sports medicine physician, because the only way to produce revenue as a physician is with your time. This cost measured in time of doing business as a team physician can be high. Unless being a team physician is very rewarding to you through personal satisfaction or the other intangible indirect benefits associated with the role, being a team physician may not be a good financial decision for you as a person and a physician, or for your practice and your family.

Teaching is one of the primary responsibilities of the team physician. After all, teaching and medicine are inseparable. Educating others is a challenging yet essential role of a team physician, and understanding the educational opportunities, responsibilities, and methods of creating a learning environment are essential qualities of the team physician. The successful teaching team physician is the one who accepts his role as an educator, understands the importance of involvement in the educational process at all levels, and is able to create an environment conducive to student learning, while at the same time serving as a valuable resource for patients, coaches, administrators, and the public.

"Show me the money" is without question the number one reason to market and advertise. That may sound silly to say, but look at some of the advertising, and it will then be time to question and understand the thought process of those who advertise and market. In this article, the authors attempt to provide information on marketing and advertising that will help your business, and that we hope will provide some thought-provoking ideas for you to pursue that will enable you to increase your company's bottom line and "show them the money."

When addressing the politics of sports medicine, it is often helpful to obtain the advice of people who work in the trenches and who have experiences that can be of benefit to clinicians in the field or who are contemplating going into the field. The goal of this project was to obtain advice from physicians who have dealt with these political issues. It is hoped that their insights will prove helpful for physicians and others who are involved in the care of athletes, regardless of the athlete's level of the play.

Much has transpired in the world of sports medicine since Herodicus, a Thracian physician of the fifth century BC, rendered his foundational theories on the use of therapeutic exercise for the maintenance of health and the treatment of disease. Unfortunately, as basic knowledge advances, history abounds in inconsistencies in regard to the proper and most effective delivery of sports medicine. This article traces the development of sports medicine and its relation to high school, college, and Olympic sports over the last centuries, and provides glimpses into what the future of the field may hold.

EVIER
NDERS

CLINICS IN SPORTS MEDICINE

THE CLINICS ARE NOW AVAILABLE ONLINE!

Access your subscription at:
http://www.theclinics.com

CLINICS IN SPORTS MEDICINE

Foreword

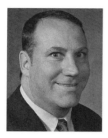

Mark D. Miller, MD

Consulting Editor

here may not be an "I" in "team," but there certainly is a "Jeff" in "Team Physician." Dr. Jeff Konin, who is a truly superlative athletic trainer and physical therapist that I have known for 4 years, has put together an outstanding issue of *Clinics in Sports Medicine*, focusing on advice for the team physician. He has assembled an all-star team of physicians, athletic trainers, and physical therapists in a no-holes-barred treatise for the Team Doc. This is a great read for team physicians at all levels of experience and for coverage of all levels of teams. Communication, politics, establishing priorities, legal and financial advice, marketing, and a whole host of issues are covered in detail. One of the more interesting articles is written by Dr. McFarland and colleagues, which provides some outstanding insight and advice from team physicians literally all over the map—lessons that have been learned the hard way, and, if closely followed, may not have to be relearned!

Jeff has certainly taught me a lot about what it takes to be a good Team Doc—I think this issue of *Clinics* has taught me even more!

Mark D. Miller, MD
Department of Orthopaedic Surgery
Division of Sports Medicine
University of Virginia Health System
P.O. Box 800753
Charlottesville, VA 22903-0753, USA

E-mail address: mdm3p@hscmail.mcc.virginia.edu

0278-5919/07/$ – see front matter
doi:10.1016/j.csm.2007.01.011
© 2007 Elsevier Inc. All rights reserved.

Clin Sports Med 26 (2007) xv–xvi

CLINICS IN SPORTS MEDICINE

Preface

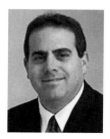

Jeff G. Konin, PhD, ATC, PT
Guest Editor

W hen Mark Miller first asked me to put together an issue revolving around the "ins and outs" behind the nonclinical roles of a team physician, I first wondered why he chose me as opposed to a team physician. After all, I don't hold a medical degree, nor have I ever served in the role of a team physician. So why ask me when there are so many others out there who have been successful team physicians and could have put this compilation together? I have known Mark Miller for nearly 5 years now, and rarely question his intuitiveness and forward-thinking. He is perhaps the ultimate multi-tasker, always performing at the highest levels of competence, and settles for nothing less than excellence. To work with him is a true pleasure and exemplifies the meaning behind the writings in this edition. It was clear to me from day 1 of our working relationship that as academically solid and clinically skilled Mark Miller is, he listens to others and understands what it takes to be successful in adapting to new environments. Together we formed a team, with contributions from many others who will never be overlooked or forgotten, that created a system of highly effective communication and trust, the two factors that I believe are necessary in any relationship. During the past 5 years, I learned a lot from Mark Miller, and I would like to believe that he learned something from me. Together, we realized more and more each day how dependant we were on each other to maintain the goals and objectives we envisioned to set the standard of care for our sports medicine department. In knowing that we are merely but one team of many that exist, we sought to glean expertise from others who have been in the trenches of all levels of sports. And so what you have is a collective product of life experiences that we believe is the first ever compiled in this format. We are so fortunate to learn from the best of the best. Anyone who has any interest in sports medicine will

0278-5919/07/$ – see front matter
doi:10.1016/j.csm.2007.01.002

© 2007 Elsevier Inc. All rights reserved.
sportsmed.theclinics.com

cherish the candid writings contained within from such highly respected individuals as Jim Andrews, Jim Whiteside, Larry Lemak, Mary Lloyd Ireland, Joel Boyd, Ed McFarland, and Freddie Fu. Whether you are a seasoned team physician or someone hoping to land a role as a future team physician, I believe that you will find the information shared in this edition to be rewarding and enjoyable reading material. I am truly honored to facilitate this less-than-scientific collection of thoughts that have more meaning and wisdom than any evidence-based study I have read to date. We should all be thankful to the individuals who have contributed their most sincere, and in many cases, controversial experiences with the rest of us. What follows is, as we always tell our students, what one will experience in the real world.

Jeff G. Konin, PhD, ATC, PT
Department of Orthopaedic Surgery
Sports Medicine and Athletic Related Trauma (SMART) Institute
College of Medicine
University of South Florida
12901 Bruce B. Downs Blvd., MDC 36
Tampa, FL 33612, USA

E-mail address: jkonin@health.usf.edu

SEVIER
UNDERS

Clin Sports Med 26 (2007) xvii

CLINICS IN SPORTS MEDICINE

Dedication

This issue of the *Clinics in Sports Medicine* is dedicated to Dan Campbell, a true friend of team physicians and many others who understood that the real meaning of sports medicine was advocating for the best interest of the athlete. Learning lessons of life from those that pass before us embodies the bond of professional and personal friendships that keep us motivated to do what we do. We will miss you Dan, but we will never forget your contributions.

Team physicians are valued members of athletic communities. To work a lifetime as a team physician requires one to possess the skills that balance one's job and personal life. At the end of every day, family and our communities come first, and our contributions to society as a whole are bigger than any sporting event. Today, we are all Hokies. Our hearts go out to the families and the Virginia Tech community affected by tragedy.

0278-5919/07/$ – see front matter
doi:10.1016/j.csm.2007.03.001

© 2007 Elsevier Inc. All rights reserved.
sportsmed.theclinics.com

Clin Sports Med 26 (2007) 137–148

CLINICS IN SPORTS MEDICINE

EVIER
NDERS

Communication: The Key to the Game

Jeff G. Konin, PhD, ATC, PT

Department of Orthopaedic Surgery, College of Medicine, University of South Florida,
12901 Bruce B. Downs Boulevard, MDC 77, Tampa, FL 33612-4766, USA

C ommunication. Communication. Communication. The author could probably stop writing this article at this point. If I did, however, you might just think my words are archaic and merely come across as yet just another cliché in a world that is overpopulated and infiltrated with acronyms and quotes to describe each and every daily encounter. So perhaps an explanation is owed to clearly justify why the word "communication" takes on a whole new level of meaning when it describes one's role as a team physician.

Many books have been published on the topic of communication, and even more courses and television shows have been presented to share with people the basics of communication. These formal teachings have focused on the characteristics related to communicating: skills such as listening, repeating one's statements for clarification, and not interrupting, just to name a few. Although these types of interventions would certainly assist one to strengthen individual communication skills, they are considered to be elementary, basic, and the bare minimum needed to develop successful communication lines when acting as team physician. Throughout the remainder of this article, the author discusses real-life communication "musts" and "tricks" that you might find to be helpful methods for successful interactions.

IMPORTANCE

Perhaps the biggest mistake one can make as a team physician as it relates to communication is to underestimate the importance of any single piece of information. The team physician must recognize at all times that he or she is a part of a team of health care providers. This means that new information regarding the injury or illness of a player must be shared with the athletic trainers and other key individuals in a timely manner. Likewise, the team physician should expect the same level of communication in return from athletic trainers. One of the most uncomfortable feelings that a medical provider associated with a team can have is to be asked a question by a coach or key person and not know the answer. It is not uncommon for coaches and others to ask the same question to

E-mail address: jeffkonin@hotmail.com

0278-5919/07/$ – see front matter
doi:10.1016/j.csm.2007.01.008
© 2007 Published by Elsevier Inc.
sportsmed.theclinics.com

multiple health care providers associated with a team, just to see if they can obtain the same response. In fact, if the question at hand pertains to a diagnosis, prognosis, or return-to-play decision, this is a common tactic that will be used by coaches in an attempt to seek out the one person on the medical team who may provide the most favorable response from the coach's perception. Be careful not to underestimate the value of each little piece of information related to a player's health, and be sure to communicate this to other appropriate medical team members. Team physicians should at all times carry telephone numbers, e-mail addresses, pagers, and any other form of communication used by medical staff members to assure timely communication.

It is absolutely critical that the team physician, and any other medical staff member for that matter, does not "grandstand" and feel compelled to be the one to deliver news that other pertinent medical staff members do not have. Feeling the need to set one's own a priori information dissemination agenda will only lead to a distrustful and uncomfortable environment. Furthermore, this has the dangerous potential of providing coaches and others with credible information that some involved medical staff members do not have. There is no place for such behavior when a team of medical providers are expected to work as one.

To avoid confusion, misinformation, and communicating through inappropriate channels, it is imperative to first identify a single person who will be the voice of the medical staff. All information regarding the health status of a player should be conveyed through this one individual. Doing this clearly lets everyone know who the reliable source of health information is. This could pertain to delivering daily injury reports, clarifying the postoperative status of a player, or communicating with the media. In some cases, coaches prefer that the medical staff not directly communicate with the media unless given permission. This is not something a team physician should feel concerned or even left out about. In fact, the author's experience is that providing coaches with injury or illness information and allowing them to convey it in their own words and terms, choosing how much information they choose to share openly with the media, is actually a wise choice. Coaches are also not obligated to follow the Health Insurance Portability and Accountability Act (HIPAA), making it much easier and less intrusive for them to share medical information.

CHAIN OF COMMAND

Physicians, despite their areas of practice, are by nature individuals who are perceived by the community as leaders. Rightly so, physicians have been placed in leadership positions and therefore often find themselves in key decision-making circumstances. Whether it be operating a private practice, serving as the chair of orthopedics for a university, or simply possessing the highest recognized health care delivery degree, physicians have come accustomed to certain privileges of respect, access, and worth. The athletic training room provides for a unique environment, one that transforms a typical single-patient health care delivery system into a multidimensional approach to caring for an entire team simultaneously. Though this may seem like a disorganized environment, the majority of these facilities are extremely organized, and the individuals working in them, especially those in director roles, know exactly how to manage all that is happening. It is the responsibility of the team physician to learn how to blend into such an environment, as opposed to visiting during random or even planned times and expecting operations to be restructured or changed during such a visit.

Just as the facility has a method of operating that contributes to its efficiency and success, each athletic team, program, or organization will have an expected communication chain of command. These will vary from program to program, sometimes making it difficult for medical staff to follow a consistent procedure. Working with one team, for example a professional organization, allows for established clear pathways of the communication chain. If one is serving as a team physician in a university setting, however, coaches from different teams may want to be notified of information in different manners. This poses a challenge to the team physician. It is imperative in all circumstances, regardless of setting, to clearly know the chain of command. Typically, the director of sports medicine, head athletic trainer, or whoever is most involved on a daily basis interacting with the athletes, coaches, and other affiliated personnel tends to have the best knowledge of how communication should be handled in varying circumstances.

Oftentimes the chain of command is tested, and puts one in an awkward situation. Regardless, the chain must be respected at all times. How does this occur? Well, you might find yourself being unexpectedly cornered by an organization's administrator. This could be an athletic director for a high school or college, a president or vice president for a university, a general manager or owner for a professional team. The question is posed to you about the status of a recently injured player. You know what the latest details are, but you haven't yet had a chance to convey this to the rest of the medical team, nor to the player himself. Do you tell what you know? Do you tell the truth and say you know the answer but it is not appropriate to share with this person first? Or do you pretend that you don't know the answer yet and then share the information with the athlete and medical staff, only to run the risk of finding out the administrator could be right behind you mingling in the training room while you are sharing the information?

There may not be a right or wrong answer to the posed questions. It may be based upon prearranged formal or informal chain-of-command procedures. For example, one setting may make it perfectly clear that regardless of the circumstances and who inquires, no information is shared until those who need to know first are informed, and those who will ultimately be informed are informed in a timely manner through appropriate means. Yet in another setting, it may be understood that certain individuals will be given courtesy information so long as it doesn't violate any privacy provisions. In such a case, once such a discussion occurs, it is the responsibility of the team physician to immediately inform members of the medical staff, so they do not get caught up in telling a different story to the same individual. This is a clear example of when planned communication patterns are as important as making appropriate medical decisions.

SUCCESSFUL METHODS

Talking about how important communication is seems somewhat elementary. Why write about how someone with a medical degree needs to learn to communicate? The answer is that it is necessary because the role of a team physician is not taught in medical school. The environment is like no other, and being an authoritative figure when present, yet being present for a small percentage of time that the actual operations carry on requires tremendous communication skills to remain informed of all issues.

There are a number of techniques that can facilitate ongoing successful communication between the team physician and the medical staff. None of these are necessarily better than the other, but by using each of them when appropriate one has a much greater chance of preventing miscommunication scenarios. In all cases, remember that communication is always a two-way street at a minimum, and most likely it will involve more than two parties. You should expect that different scenarios will be facilitated by different individuals, and that it will not always be a single person's responsibility to initiate all communications. As such, every person with a vested interest in this process must be familiar with protocol and follow it consistently.

Having discussed ad nauseam the need for thorough and timely communication, how does one determine what constitutes "important" information? Of course without any prior agreed- upon set of circumstances, it is always left up to the discretion of each individual. Doesn't this seem like a risky way to operate with such critical consequences at stake? In the author's opinion, it is extremely risky. As a result of this, when I was in the position of director of sports medicine, I provided some written guidelines for all staff to follow, so that we at least had some sense of understanding the type of information that I deemed the most timely and important. The following are what we used as standing requests for communication with the director of sports medicine (DSM):

1. Information on any student-athlete who has been admitted to a hospital should be conveyed to the DSM immediately.
2. Information on any student-athlete who has been referred to a medical specialist on or off-campus should be conveyed to the DSM within 24 hours.
3. Information on any student-athlete who is being referred for imaging or laboratory work should be conveyed to the DSM within 24 hours.
4. Results from an image test, laboratory work, or medical specialist consultation should be conveyed to the DSM immediately.
5. Information on any student-athlete who has been entered into the crisis management plan should be conveyed to the DSM immediately, if in the judgment of the referring individual the person is in a position to do harm to oneself or others.

6. Any student-athlete who has not seen improvement in his or her rehabilitation plan after 2 weeks of intervention should receive a consult from the DSM.
7. Any-student athlete who receives a consult by the DSM should have a progress report conveyed to the DSM.
8. Any student-athlete who has an uncertain acute injury should receive a second opinion from another certified athletic trainer (ATC) before any random treatment intervention approach.
9. Any student athlete or coach who has concerns about the delivery of sports medicine should be referred to the DSM.

Although this list may not be all-inclusive, it provides for a clear understanding of what constitutes immediate communication in an effort to stay abreast of circumstances, as well as to head off potential concerns. There is no doubt that some individuals will read this list and think that it is a form of over communicating or micromanaging; however, it is always far better to over communicate than to have no clear understanding of what type of information needs to be shared.

There is another intangible that comes into play and that is often overlooked by medical staff personnel, yet is considered by many to be immensely important. Just as a director of sports medicine wants to be informed by other staff members of critical circumstances, so too do the director's supervisors. In some cases, the desire is merely to be kept abreast of issues of greater concern. For example, it is not likely that the athletic director needs to know that an athlete is going to get blood work performed; however, if an athlete was rushed to an emergency room, or had a major surgery performed, then often administrators and others want to be informed from a caring perspective, not necessarily merely from an administrative perspective, although the two may blend. An example of this might occur if you as a team physician were caring for an athlete from a small college who either just underwent surgery or was hospitalized for a medical illness. Despite the fact that the condition itself may appear routine to you, such as a successful appendectomy, it is not so common to the athlete who has never experienced this before. Add to this that the athlete hails from the other side of the country, and has no immediate family members nearby. In cases like these, college officials will want to make it a point to support the individual beyond what might be normally expected. This could involve officials taking turns visiting the athlete in the hospital, and also keeping in constant contact with the athlete's family to inform them on a regular basis of her condition. You can imagine how important such communication would be to a family under these circumstances, and you can also appreciate how critical it is for everyone to be on the same page with timely information to share regarding the status of the athlete. Again, it is always important to have a protocol so people know who the "go-to" person is for accurate information.

If you are working with an organization such as a professional sports teams or a university that has a formal media or public relations department, you want to be very clear on your role and the mechanism for communicating information with such individuals. Remember, the media, whether affiliated with your program or serving in an external role for a local newspaper, have a job to do that involves disseminating information to the public. Regardless of the information that is sought, you should never lose sight of the fact that you will be a part of an established protocol of how and when to share information. You may want to assist these people in many ways, and there is nothing wrong with that philosophy, but always follow established protocol. Perhaps the greatest motivation to share such information with media stems from the concern for providing accurate information. Medical personnel often complain about being misquoted or seeing inappropriate terms used to display information to the general public. Yes, it is frustrating. The author believes that there are a few tips you can use to avoid such concerns.

First, always speak with one voice. No matter who is summoned by request from the media, always refer them to the same person on the medical staff for comment. In some cases, this may not even happen, because you may choose or be directed by a coach not to comment at all. This is not such a bad thing, because you will never be misquoted under these guidelines! Second, avoid as best you can impromptu, hallway type conversations. You will be quoted, and you won't remember exactly what you said to who in a passing moment. Going back to the go-to person approach, let one voice speak, and better yet, let one voice write. The key to avoid being misquoted or accused of providing information in an inappropriate manner is to only share information in a written form when allowed. You should always maintain a file for your own records of the information you provide, and you may want to concurrently send copies of your information sharing to those who you think might need to be informed of your contact with media. Last, remember that the media, especially those who work for your organization, can be very helpful. Crafting proactive press releases and translating medical terminology into laymen's terms can help reduce questions and concerns that may arise relating to an injured athlete.

PRACTICAL FORMS OF COMMUNICATION

Today we live in an era of high-speed technology. Combine this with the "I need to know yesterday" mentality of those working in athletics, and you are faced with a challenge to communicate in a thorough and timely manner. Whether or not you agree with the sense of urgency is irrelevant. It is your responsibility to figure out how to meet the expectations of those you are in a supportive role for. Again, egos must be pushed aside, and expected authoritative behaviors have no place in the world of being a team physician. The author remembers vividly having a team physician tell me once that he would communicate how and when he felt like it with me regarding any athlete's injury status. You can only imagine the thoughts that raced through my mind as I was trying to build a team of collaborative individuals who shared the same vision of providing the highest standard of care. I struggled to identify how we could transform this type of an approach by the team physician into our goals, and each time I realized that the individual was not familiar enough with the expectations of the organization; he was merely one small piece of the much bigger picture. There is no place for individual demands of communication tactics that do not coincide with a team's or organization's needs. Remember, everyone is replaceable. If you are unable to meet the needs of an organization, then you may not be the best fit for that group at that particular time. They are the customers, and they will choose the product that best fits their needs. If you know ahead of time that your schedule might be conflicting with event coverage and clinic visits, that your method of communication is much different then they expect, or that there is any other issue that might prevent you from being the total team player in your role, you have an obligation to openly communicate this. You must compromise to an acceptable position as best you can, or recognize that your inability to meet the organization's needs must force you to pass up the role.

Now back to the technology era. Aside from maintaining written records for any historical or legal reason, sharing timely information in the form of a formal memorandum has become obsolete. Dictated and transcribed documents that are prepared and copied to appropriate personnel are filed, and usually received at a time much later than the news needs to be shared. Although there is a place for such documentation, on most occasions the paperwork is seen as follow-up documentation and filed in one's records.

There is no doubt that direct person-to-person communication is best. Absent a face-to-face contact, the telephone is the quickest and most efficient mechanism for conveying information. Cell phones and beepers are a must, and any other form of mobile communication serves as a safe conduit to locate individuals. There is a haunting expectation in the eyes of some that team physicians are on call 24 hours a day, 7 days a week. In fact, this is the very reason that some physicians choose not to be associated with athletic teams! This expectation is not untrue, but again, it is imperative that you set parameters from the beginning regarding what type of communication is expected. Perhaps you don't want to be called in the middle of each night with athletic injury related issues; however, if there were an injury or illness that rose to the level of an emergency, would you not want to be informed in a timely manner, because you are the person ultimately responsible for the medical care in the role of team physician? The key here is to know as a team of medical professionals how "timely" is defined, and what circumstances warrant your immediate knowledge and awareness. Absent a clear understanding of the medical team, as well as of coaches, players, and administrators, you can expect numerous calls at all times of the day regarding all topics and issues, ranging from emergencies that should be managed through quicker and more appropriate channels to favors from the assistant coach asking for you to give his aunt Edna advice for her arthritic knee.

Electronic mail (e-mail) can be a very effective form of communication so long as both parties are able to access the information within the time frame you wish for them to see it. If the matter is of some urgency, you may not be guaranteed they are in a location or position to access e-mail. This may be because of poor reception or because they are in a meeting where it would be rude to view and respond to e-mails. Thus timing may be a small issue. If, however, your intent through an e-mail is merely to provide an "FYI" pertaining to an issue, reading the message when convenient allows for a great way to share updates without being time-consuming. This holds especially true if you wish to inform more than one person at a time; e-mail can be much more efficient than making numerous phone calls. The author must add a disclaimer here. Anything you put in writing through an e-mail is an official document, subject to viewing by others, and more importantly, subject to either purposeful or accidental forwarding to individuals not meant to see the original e-mail. The author is sure that each and every one of you has experienced an inadvertently sent e-mail. Perhaps you were the recipient and it widened your eyes, or perhaps you hit the send button accidentally to the wrong person and you encountered that empty feeling in your stomach. Regardless, there is high risk associated with e-mail communication. You should always be professional, careful as to what you write and how you write e-mails, and always make sure that the information you are sharing follows appropriate legal guidelines for security and privacy. Carbon copies ("cc's") and blind carbon copies ("bcc's"), which are inappropriate and outdated terms relative to a computer file, are also ways to provide information to some without others knowing; however, these run an additional risk that one needs to always keep in mind. I have seen people who were bcc'd for courtesy purposes not pay attention and reply to all, only to let others on to the fact they were originally bcc'd in the first e-mail, appearing as though the sender was hiding their involvement. Every form of communication comes with a risk, and you should never underestimate the potential for carelessness.

COMMON COMMUNICATION PITFALLS OF TEAM PHYSICIANS

The author is no David Letterman, and I have surely made my share of communication mistakes over the course of my professional career. In no particular order, here are the top ten communication mistakes that I see team physicians falling prey to.

Not Communicating at All

Without a doubt the absence of communication is the ultimate pitfall of a successful team approach to speaking with one voice. If you choose to establish your own form of communication and it leans toward minimizing information sharing, you will be initiating your own eventual demise as a team physician.

Not Communicating Enough

Less than expected communication is almost as dangerous as no communication at all. With no communication, others know what to expect or not expect from you, and they know they will have to track you down on all cases for information. When you inconsistently communicate, it is like making others play a game of roulette, not knowing when you even have information that is relevant to share. This is dangerous, and thus the importance of having established expectations for communication clearly delineated and agreed upon ahead of time.

Not Acknowledging Communication

Leaving a voice mail or e-mail, or even sending written memos, does not confirm that the recipient has successfully received the information. One can't assume that by merely sending information that is has been received. It is courtesy to reply even in the simplest forms to acknowledge receipt and to minimize any questions as to whether you have been informed.

Careless E-mails

Inadvertently sending e-mails to those who you did not intend to see what you wrote is rather difficult to backtrack from. Furthermore, be careful in short, abrupt e-mail replies and other statements made. Unfortunately, the intent of your tone can be misinterpreted as being negative, and even brash. The very nature of using quick, short responses to be efficient has a tendency of being perceived by others as non-empathetic, impatient, and even condescending at times. Bottom line—e-mail does not convey a personality!

Bad Day of Communicating

How many times have you heard the phrase, "He is just having a bad day"? As a team physician, there is no place for bad days or bad interactions. Remember, you are working with a team, so one bad interaction spreads through dozens of others within minutes, and your reputation, interest, bedside manner, and other characteristics will be seen from a negative light from there on. Two bad interactions with athletes from two different teams in a high school or collegiate setting now double the negative publicity of the perception that they have for you. There is no magic equation to strive for, no matter how many positive interactions you have, none can reverse the damage of a negative one. The author might even go as far as to say that if your bad day involves a coach or administrator, you have done more harm for yourself than you can possibly imagine.

Not Recognizing the Importance of Communication

The author can't emphasize this point enough. Consider this scenario: you receive a phone call in your office from the parent of an athlete who you performed recent surgery on. The athlete is having small setbacks in rehabilitation progress, and the parent is concerned. Of course, with permission from the athlete if over 18 years of age, you speak to the concerned parent and convey your thoughts. You are concerned that you have reached a peak with conservative care, and perhaps another intervention is necessary, possibly even another surgery. Seems like a normal everyday telephone conversation you may encounter; however, you do not inform the athletic trainer of this telephone interaction. Later in the day, the athlete or the parents ask the athletic trainer similar questions that were posed to you. The athletic trainer's response is that the athlete is still progressing well despite the setback, and that there are no immediate plans for another surgical intervention. Now the parents and the athlete are confused, and either the athletic trainer or the physician will lose credibility, and you will need to spend more time clarifying the appropriate status and prognosis to the point where you are believed and trusted by the athlete and the parents. This is an all too common happening that is 100% avoidable with a quick call.

Not Being a Chameleon

Working as a team physician for an organization like a high school or college, where you are responsible for caring for a multitude of athletes representing male and female sports of all kinds, can be a challenging factor in communication. With respect to health care, certainly everyone must be treated equally and fairly; however, with respect to communication, there must be an opposite approach. How so, you ask? Simply put, when examining an athlete and ultimately delivering news, especially news that will not be perceived as positive, one must know the individual well enough to understand and predict how he or she will react to your message. Maybe you need to palpate firm and deep to assess a tissue structure. This might be fine with a 300-pound linemen who won't blink when you perform the task. But to the 95-pound female cross country runner who is experiencing excruciating pain in her lower limb, there may be no level of acceptable sensitive palpation that you could use to prevent her from breaking down emotionally from the pain and overall discomfort of the experience. Always be cognizant of your athlete's personality characteristics, what sport he or she plays, something about the sport, and where this injury falls with respect to the competitive season. Never ask when the next important game is! To a competitive athlete, there is no off-season and no day off! A bad memory is not a good thing, so don't pretend to remember things about the athletes to impress them. Use the sports medicine staff for as much of a debriefing as you can obtain before each interaction with an athlete, much the same way that you would do in a private clinical practice by reading a patient's medical chart before entering the patient's room. Demonstrating to athletes that you do not remember them, their injury, their sport, and so forth, will instantaneously depreciate your credibility in their eyes.

Bypassing Chains of Communication

Perhaps this is one of those informal rules that you never see written other than in the standardized organizational chart seen in every policy and procedure manual. Yet, there is a reason reporting lines are established and adhered to. Simply put, they contribute to appropriate types of information being funneled to necessary individuals and levels. There is no need to impress others of higher administrative levels of your knowledge, and less of a reason to share information with those that have no right to be informed of confidential information. The best piece of advice the author can give here is to understand that most athletic directors have the highest level of trust and confidence in their directors of sports medicine. Athletic directors are in the business of raising large sums of money, and operating in many cases with upwards of tens of millions of dollars in a budget for their programs. They are not in the business of sports medicine, and they clearly acknowledge that. To them sports medicine plays a supportive role, along with many other supportive areas that all lead to a successful athletic program and organization. Therefore, athletic directors lean to their sports medicine director when issues arise in this area. Any topic you or others bring to an athletic director will likely land back on the desk of the sports medicine director. Never underestimate the bond of trust if you are an outsider looking in. Most people on the outside looking in do not understand or appreciate the inner workings of an athletic program, and very commonly demonstrate such lack of knowledge with the simplest statements and ideas they suggest. Respect people's roles at all times.

Not Knowing Clinical Policies

Not knowing clinical policies is a formula for litigation. Not only should you as a team physician be familiar with policies that relate to concussion management, emergency action plans for all venues, environmental illnesses such as dehydration, return-to-play criteria, pharmacology, and others, you must also be heavily invested in the development and approval of each policy. In the majority of cases, you are the individual most responsible for medical decisions. Take an interest in these policies, and use the strengths of the staff and other experts who can assist you in developing the most reasonable policies for the program you work with given the resources available, and be sure to follow accepted national guidelines, evidence-based approaches, and community standards. If done correctly, this process cannot only demonstrate a meaningful vehicle for forced communication, it can also lead to the justification for additional needed resources such as automated external defibrillators, transportation vehicles, and other critical items often left out solely for budgetary reasons.

Don't Freely Gossip

Being a team physician comes with some celebrity status. The author does not think that it matters if you are the team physician for a professional team or the local high school. Either way, you are a prominent figure and play a critical decision-making role that everybody else in that environment yields to. You are vulnerable to numerous casual conversations in passing through life's daily chores. When you get a haircut, if you happen to shop for groceries on the way home from work, if you are eating lunch at the country club, people with curious minds will prompt you for answers regarding athlete's injuries. You must remain loyal to the very same principles of privacy, confidentiality, and chain of command as if you were in the work setting. These passing informal encounters will never cease, but your professional and polite affirmation that it would be inappropriate for you to comment will ultimately resonate with the repeat offenders, and should reduce the number of inquiries over time.

SUMMARY

Being a team physician requires a whole new set of communications skills, depending on the organization that one is affiliated with. There may be a single expected procedure to follow, or multiple procedures may be required to meet the needs of various organizations. Regardless, it is imperative for the team physician to understand that his or her role is vital to those who seek accurate and timely information, thus potentially requiring physicians to adapt their current methods for communicating. Learning how to communicate as a team physician in a timely and accurate manner, understanding the appropriate chain of command, and avoiding common pitfalls associated with improper and sometimes adverse forms of communication will pave the way for an excellent long-term working relationship.

Clin Sports Med 26 (2007) 149–160

CLINICS IN SPORTS MEDICINE

EVIER
NDERS

Accessibility of the Team Physician

Tom Kuster, MS, ATC, NASM-PES[a],*, David Knitter, MD[a,b],
Lenny Navitskis, Med, ATC, CSCS, NREMT-I[c]

[a]Department of Sports Medicine, MSC 2301, James Madison University,
Godwin 128, Harrisonburg, VA 22807, USA
[b]Center for Innovation in Health and Human Services, Department of Health Sciences,
MSC 4301, James Madison University, Harrisonburg, VA 22807, USA
[c]Department of Sports Medicine, University of Georgia Athletic Association, P.O. Box 1472,
Athens, GA 30603-1472, USA

T he transition to the care of the college student-athlete carries with it a number of adjustments. In private practice it is customary to make medical decisions and initiate therapies from the confines of the examination room. The doctor-patient relationship is the principal focus. Although this relationship remains paramount in college athletics, the world of concerned and affected parties dramatically expands. It is in this context that the authors explore the concept of access in the role of a team physician. To use what is becoming an over used cliché, what makes one a valued team physician is being "the right person, in the right place at the right time." The transition to the care of the college student-athlete carries with it a number of adjustments. In private practice it is customary to make medical decisions and initiate therapies from the confines of the examination room. The doctor-patient relationship is the principal focus. Although this relationship remains paramount in college athletics, the world of concerned and affected parties dramatically expands. It is in this context that the authors explore the concept of access in the role of a team physician. To use what is becoming an over used cliché, what makes one a valued team physician is being "the right person, in the right place at the right time."

WHAT IS ACCESSIBILITY?

The first question one must address regarding access is from whose perspective are we viewing the team physician? For the athlete, accessibility may mean that the team physician's hours or office location do not conflict with class or practice schedules. For the athletic trainer, the key features of access may be the availability of the team physician during athletic events, during off hours, or while the team is traveling. For the coach, access focuses on the most rapid

*Corresponding author. E-mail address: kustertj@jmu.edu (T. Kuster).

0278-5919/07/$ – see front matter   © 2007 Elsevier Inc. All rights reserved.
doi:10.1016/j.csm.2006.12.001   sportsmed.theclinics.com

return to full health and active participation of the athlete. For the parent, access implies timely communication of treatment or testing on their son or daughter, who is often quite some distance from home. For the team physician, access issues surround the impact of the athletics responsibilities on his or her other patient care responsibilities or family. For the athletics administrator, access results in all of the above parties feeling as if their needs are being met. As one looks at institutions, even within the relatively homogenous realm of college athletics, it is readily apparent that there are many solutions to the problem of defining and using the services of the team physician.

ROLE AND RESPONSIBILITY OF THE TEAM PHYSICIAN

As we look at the value of accessibility, it is important to examine the varied roles of the team physician within a defined set of core duties:

- Patient care
    Scope of practice
    Pre-participation examination
    Illnesses and injuries
    Event coverage
- Medical resource and health policy advocate
    Policies and procedures
    Off-hour or off-location consults
- Medical liaison and specialty provider access

PATIENT CARE

Scope of Practice

Despite the existence of sports medicine as a recognized subspecialty certification by the American Board of Internal Medicine, there is surprisingly little in the literature about the types of conditions encountered by a team physician [1,2]. In fact, the only published article chronicles the experience of Steiner and colleagues' experience at Harvard University [3]. In the Harvard study, 79% of the evaluations over a 2-year period were related to musculoskeletal complaints. A response to this perception is that the designated team physician is often an orthopedic surgeon. General medical problems are referred to the college health center. As we delve deeper into the complexities of accessibility, this practice brings with it a potential for perpetuating the perception that non-musculoskeletal conditions have a lesser contribution to the overall health of the college student-athlete.

In reviewing the unpublished data of the authors' institution, covering more than 600 athletes in 28 men's and women's sports in Division I-AA, one will find a decidedly different picture. At James Madison University, we have a weekday general medical clinic covered by the team physician and an orthopedic clinic covered by our contracting team orthopedist 2 or 3 days per week.

Table 1 summarizes the usage of only the general medical clinic. In comparison with the Harvard data there is considerable difference in the rate of overall use of resources: 0.9 visits per capita at Harvard compared with James Madison University's 3.7 visits per capita.

Table 1
Usage of the general medical clinic

Sport	Gender	Total visits 2005–06	Total visits 2004–05	Roster 2005–06	Roster 2004–05	Visits/capita 2005–06	Visits/capita 2004–05	Change
Archery	Both	40	12	19	19	2.1	0.6	107.7%
Baseball	Men's	114	85	30	28	3.8	3.0	22.4%
Basketball	Men's	79	68	13	14	6.1	4.9	22.3%
Basketball	Women's	55	112	18	13	3.1	8.6	−95.3%
Cheerleading	Both	16	12	30	30	0.5	0.4	28.6%
Diving	Men's	12	33	3	3	4.0	11.0	−93.3%
Diving	Women's	9	5	3	2	3.0	2.5	18.2%
Fencing	Both	28	16	7	7	4.0	2.3	54.5%
Field hockey	Women's	64	68	23	24	2.8	2.8	−1.8%
Football	Men's	195	178	94	99	2.1	1.8	14.3%
Golf	Men's	5	2	8	5	0.6	0.4	43.9%
Golf	Women's	10	7	8	6	1.3	1.2	6.9%
Gymnastics	Men's	71	50	11	8	6.5	6.3	3.2%
Gymnastics	Women's	76	96	24	22	3.2	4.4	−31.8%
Lacrosse	Women's	108	144	25	25	4.3	5.8	−28.6%
Soccer	Men's	143	82	24	33	6.0	2.5	82.3%
Soccer	Women's	141	92	31	25	4.5	3.7	21.1%
Softball	Women's	147	78	18	19	8.2	4.1	66.2%
Swimming	Men's	77	67	23	17	3.3	3.9	−16.3%
Swimming	Women's	126	116	22	19	5.7	6.1	−6.4%
Tennis	Men's	14	10	9	9	1.6	1.1	33.3%
Tennis	Women's	10	10	8	5	1.3	2.0	−46.2%
Track CC	Men's	66	68	81	42	0.8	1.6	−66.1%
Track CC	Women's	215	137	58	34	3.7	4.0	−8.3%
Volleyball	Women's	119	62	19	15	6.3	4.1	41.0%
Wrestling	Men's	198	183	28	28	7.1	6.5	7.9%
Totals		2138	1793	637	551	3.7	3.7	—

As you can see from Table 2, the categories for evaluation differed. Ear, nose and throat disorders were the most common complaint, with musculoskeletal injuries playing a much smaller role at 16.5%.

Although the data have not been tabulated by sport, athlete, or complaint, there were 479 visits to our orthopedic clinic during the 2005–06 academic year. As you can see from Table 3, even with the addition of the orthopedic clinic data, the majority of our physician related visits were non-musculoskeletal in nature.

From Table 4 one can see that the majority of the visits to the general medical clinic were for initial evaluation. This data is consistent with the non-musculoskeletal average from the Harvard study, and consistent with the notion that the majority of physician encounters are related to acute or self-limited conditions [3].

Table 5 demonstrates a summary of the breakdown by category and visit type and gender. As might be anticipated, categories associated with more chronic conditions (ie, asthma, dysmenorrhea, endocrine and rheumatologic disorders) tended to have a higher rate of follow-up, and those with a more acute nature (ie, gastroenteritis) had a lower rate of follow-up. The distribution between the sexes reveal several notable trends, with a low female ratio in concussion evaluations, minor surgeries, and dermatologic disorders (ie, conta-gious skin lesions in competitive wrestling) and a female preponderance in endocrine, gynecologic, hematologic, and rheumatologic conditions.

Full exploration of the reasons for the differences in quantity and scope of use between the authors' institution and the Harvard study are beyond the scope of this article. One possible explanation, however, may be more open access to a general medical physician. An observation from the informal survey of our conference institutions was that those who used a general medical resource away from the athletic training room (ie, university health centers) tended to perceive general medical conditions as uncommon occurrences in their student athlete populations. This is in contrast to our situation, in which the general medical clinic is located at a location central to our athletic training facilities.

As venues have become more geographically diverse, one would anticipate that this would potentially influence the use those teams made of the services of the team physician. Currently our institution has three athletic training room facilities. One that houses the majority of our sports is also the location of the general medical clinic. A second is located a short walking distance away (city equivalent of two or three blocks) in a facility that houses the football, field hockey, lacrosse, and cheerleading athletic trainers. A third more distant facility (roughly six to eight blocks) houses the men's and women's basketball teams. As can be seen from Fig. 1, location appears to have little influence on the use of the general medical clinic, with the most distant teams having the highest rate of use.

Another observation is that moving from one facility to another also seems to have little bearing on the rates of use. The 2005–06 school year marked the

Table 2

Conditions seen in the general medical clinic

	Visits 2005–06	% Total
Allergy	40	1.9%
Cardiac	32	1.5%
Concussion	85	4.0%
Dermatology	143	6.7%
Endocrine	14	0.7%
Ear, nose, throat disorders	491	23.0%
Gastrointestinal	122	5.7%
Genitourinary	25	1.2%
Gynecological	30	1.4%
Hematology	21	1.0%
Infections	345	16.1%
Miscellaneous	63	2.9%
Musculoskeletal	352	16.5%
Neuropsychological	98	4.6%
Pulmonary	140	6.6%
Rheumatology	18	0.8%
Minor surgery	118	5.5%
Totals	2137	100.0%

opening of the "near" athletic training room. This resulted in the movement of teams previously served by the central athletic training room. As you can see from Table 1, the per capita use rates of these teams were not changed by this transition. The exception to this observation is a 28.6% reduction in use by the women's lacrosse team. Upon further analysis, it appears that this reduction was more a consequence of a change in practice time of the lacrosse team that coincided with the scheduled hours of the general medical clinic. Even with the change, this team remained an above-average (4.7 visits per capita) user of medical services.

Pre-participation Examination

Improving the perception of accessibility to the team physician begins with the introduction of the athlete to the medical care system. This relationship can best begin with the pre-participation examination. Although this encounter is brief, it gives the team physician the opportunity to meet with all the athletes on a yearly basis. Athletes who have special needs or ongoing health issues can be identified and arrangements for follow up recommended. Although the pre-participation examination is an essential requirement for all first year

Table 3

Orthopedic clinic and general medical clinic visits

Musculosketal	831	31.8%
Non-musculoskeletal	1785	68.2%
Total	2616	100%

Table 4
Types of visits to the general medical clinic

Gender	Visit type		Total	% Total
	Initial	Follow up	Total	% Total
Men's	724	278	1002	46.9%
Women's	826	309	1135	53.1%
Total	1551	587	2138	—
% Total	72.5%	27.5%	—	—

and transfer athletes, it can also be a useful tool in identifying off-season injuries or changes in previous borderline medical conditions.

The pre-participation examination can also go a long way in the establishment of trust and communication among the team physician, the athlete, the sports medicine staff, and members of the coaching staff. For an incoming freshman athlete, this first encounter may very well be the most intensive physical he or she has ever experienced. The student-athlete will undoubtedly ask questions throughout the process, and it is the responsibility of the team physician to provide answers and information in understandable terms. For the sports medicine staff, this examination provides a baseline assessment of the athlete's health that will be followed for the next 4 to 5 years. Communication amongst the sports medicine team is essential. Without proper communication and attention to detail, the sports medicine team is susceptible to lack of trust and loss of confidence from athletes and coaches. Although it is recognized as

Table 5
Visit type category and gender breakdown

Category	% Initial	% Female
Allergy	75.0%	52.5%
Cardiac	78.1%	81.3%
Concussion	77.6%	35.3%
Dermatology	60.8%	37.8%
Endocrine	50.0%	92.9%
Ear, nose, throat disorders	71.5%	55.0%
Gastrointestinal	82.8%	65.6%
Genitourinary	64.0%	64.0%
Gynecologic	60.0%	100.0%
Hematologic	71.4%	90.5%
Infectious	78.9%	46.8%
Miscellaneous	69.8%	52.4%
Musculoskeletal	71.9%	52.0%
Neurologic	71.4%	56.1%
Pulmonary	69.3%	61.4%
Rheumatologic	66.7%	88.9%
Minor surgery	72.9%	35.6%
Total	72.5%	53.1%

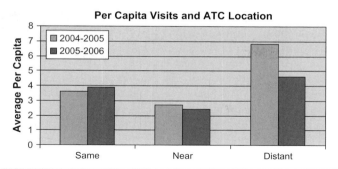

Fig. 1. General medical clinic usage.

a medical necessity, the pre-participation examination can also be viewed as a valuable public relations tool for the team physician.

Injury and Illness

As with any resource available, the physical accessibility of the team physician to the athletic system will in large part determine the extent to which his or her services are used. Once an illness reaches a certain critical threshold, medical attention will be sought no matter what the perceived obstacles. The location of the team physician will significantly influence the perception of accessibility. Rather than simply being seen at athletic events, the physician who holds clinics at location and times that are best conducive to the student athlete's attendance will greatly enhance overall accessibility. The authors have seen this at our institution, and believe it may explain why the use of the general medical clinic differs so greatly from that in published studies. When asked why they presented to clinic on this specific occasion, athletes in many instances responded that they were "passing by" or that the coach wanted them "checked out" before practice.

This emphasizes the second critical aspect of improving accessibility: the timing of clinic hours. As is presented by the authors' current data, the per capita rate of physician interactions has dramatically increased. In reviewing the exit interviews of the student athletes, the reason for this shift was readily apparent. The previous system contracted with a general practitioner in the community who scheduled clinic hours before his private practice office hours. Athletes who developed conditions requiring medical attention outside of the morning clinic hours were worked into the physician's office practice, located some distance from campus. With the restructuring, the clinic was held in the early afternoon. Although there was only a twofold to threefold increase in the hours of the clinic, there was a 10 fold increase in per capita use. Class schedules and practice times tend to take precedence over health concerns. By mitigating this barrier in structuring the clinic hours in the relative lull between these two periods, earlier detection and treatment of medical conditions was facilitated. As was observed in the previous section with our women's lacrosse team, there is no ideal schedule for clinic hours, but one that results from a compromise between athlete and physician availability works best.

A secondary aspect that improves the visibility of the team physician is a consistent schedule. As an experiment tested at our institution in the first year after restructuring, we held the clinic at different times on different days to better accommodate the athlete schedules. The result was daily confusion as to when the clinic would be held, despite the publication and dissemination of this information to all parties. A more optimal compromise at our institution was a consistent time during the week, with exceptions handled on a case-by-case basis.

Event Coverage

Given the absence of monetary or time constraints, most coaches would not object to the team physician being present at all their major events. Although the potential for injury exists for all sports, the reality is that the inherent risk of some sports is significantly greater than others. Again, one must make a compromise over what events the team physician will be present. In an informal survey of the sports medicine departments in our conferences, sports that were covered by a physician varied. In general, covered sports fell into two categories:

- Those that involve recurring high-impact collisions
  Football
  Ice hockey
  Lacrosse
- Those that have potential for such collisions
  Basketball
  Gymnastics
  Soccer
  Diving
  Wrestling

From review of the authors' own data from the 2005-06 academic year presented in Fig. 2, the proposed distribution of coverage appears to be justified. A secondary factor complicating treatment decisions is that many of the concussion evaluations resulted from injuries incurred during practice settings, or from injuries outside of athletics. Given the varied make-up of the athletics departments surveyed, this list is a compilation of the sports covered, with differing institutional decisions for similar sports. There is also the added requirement for coverage at institution-sponsored conference or National Collegiate Athletic Association (NCAA) events.

MEDICAL RESOURCE AND HEALTH POLICY ADVOCATE

Policies and Procedures

A core responsibility of the team physician is an active involvement in the formation and review of institutional policies. In many instances, the team physician serves as the institution's athletic medical director. The higher the

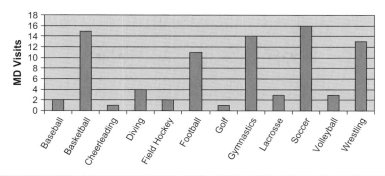

Fig. 2. MD visits per athletic team.

likelihood that an athletic trainer has to make a judgment that may be construed as a medical decision, the greater the importance that the team physician be involved in the creation of that policy. In keeping with the previous discussion of physician coverage, the concussion policy is a prime example. Concussions occasionally occur in sports with a low inherent risk, and return-to-competition decisions may need to be made without the input of a team physician. In creating a written policy with clearly defined return-to-competition criteria, both the athletic trainer and the team physician are protected. Unfortunate examples in which adverse outcomes resulted from lack of institutional policy or failure to follow said policy are not unknown.

One must be careful to not misconstrue the establishment of written policy and procedure with the creation of standing orders. Statements by the National Athletic Trainers Association (NATA) recognize the initial assessment of a concussed athlete, when a team physician is not available, as within the scope of practice of an athletic trainer [4]. Standing orders place the athletic trainer in the position of making a medical decision outside of the recognized scope of practice. When the team physician accessibility is limited because of time or distance constraints, there is a tendency to create protocols to speed up either the evaluation or the treatment of the athlete. At their most benign, these orders may increase the cost; however, at their worst, they delay the recognition or treatment of life-threatening conditions. In contrast to a well-researched and designed policy, standing orders increase the liability potential for both the athletic trainer and team physician.

Medical Consults

From the perspective of the athletic trainer, having access to the team physician as a medical consultant ranks higher in importance than the time the physician spends in the athletic training room. The specific role and responsibility of the team physician in any given situation should be clearly communicated in advance. Expectations should be discussed from both the physician's and athletic trainer's points of view. The physician must have a clear understanding as to the skill and comfort level of the sports medicine staff. This may take a variable amount of time to obtain, and typically the longer the relationship, the better the level of trust will be on both sides. Unfortunately, athletes have no greater degree of control over the timing of their physical symptoms than does the general population. Illnesses not infrequently peak during the hours most distant from scheduled clinic times. Therefore, the duties of triage generally fall on the shoulders of the athletic trainer. An agreed-upon level of access between the physician and athletic trainer should be both desirable and understandable.

The NATA has recognized this burden of decision, and has expanded its focus on the evaluation of and exposure to nontraumatic injuries in the academic preparation of athletic trainers. Athletic trainers need to be educated on how to recognize and communicate the most relevant signs and symptoms of nontraumatic injuries and illnesses, and also, with the aid of institutional policies, on how to recognize and guide the response to those situations that require urgent or emergent evaluations. Although the addition of these objectives is a step in the right direction, one can hope to introduce little more than basic concepts. Most of their training is by necessity on the job.

The importance of open and free communication between the athletic trainer and the team physician cannot be overemphasized. A team physician who consciously or unconsciously makes it difficult for the athletic trainer to access his medical expertise places a burden of decision-making on the athletic trainer that may result in inappropriate or delayed referrals to acute care settings. A secondary benefit of these interactions of the team physician and athletic trainer is that they create teachable moments when the evaluation and communication content flow can be improved.

It is understood that the team physician cannot be everywhere all the time. In such instances it is imperative for the team physician and sports medicine staff to have prearranged, planned access to medical services. This is also important in those situations in which the team physician does not have an on-site clinic or office. The avenues of communication between the athletic trainer and team physician need to be open. Methods of communicating can include cell phone access, e-mail, pager, and the like—the point being that the team physician needs to make every effort to provide the athletic trainer with a means of reaching him or her when the situation requires communication. It should be avoided if at all possible to require the athletic trainer to have to go through a "gatekeeper" to reach the physician. Having to speak with administrative assistants, nurses, and others rather than the physician directly only further slows down the exchange of information between the athletic trainer and physician.

MEDICAL LIAISON AND SPECIALTY PROVIDER ACCESS

A team physician who is an accessible and integrated member of the sports medicine team and who is in touch with the medical providers within the community can be a valuable resource in establishing specialty provider access. The timing of medical referrals to specialty physicians can prove paramount in the delivery of quality health care to the athlete and aid in return to competition as quickly and as safely as possible. An established relationship, through communication, service, and public relation assistance, will help maintain the efficiency of outside physician referrals and increase the overall quality of care. The sports medicine team should not wait until a specialty provider is needed. Efforts should be made to seek out potential specialty providers in the community. By establishing the relationship in advance, the sports medicine team will more often be rewarded with cooperation and convenient and simple access to providers, who genuinely want to be involved.

An accessible team physician will also be available to provide timely communication and serve as the liaison between the specialty provider, the athlete, and the sports medicine staff. As was suggested at the beginning of this article, the involved parties in the treatment of athletes extend well beyond this classic doctor-patient relationship. Coaches, parents, administrators, and even the media may wish to interpose themselves in the evaluation and treatment process. Yet despite the expanded sphere of influence, the primary responsibility of the team physician remains unchanged—the health and welfare of the athlete. The pathway to maximizing one's success toward this end is effective and timely communication.

Physicians for athletics often find themselves translating the results of testing, therapy, or consultant evaluations into a format that coaches and administrators can use to adjust for the present and future limitations of the involved athlete. Although participation in athletics does open oneself to a lesser degree of privacy than the average patient has, there are often sensitive issues that are discussed and have no direct bearing on athletic participation. A challenge to the team physician is making this discrimination while maintaining the confidence and comfort of the athlete about addressing these issues with you in the future.

And speaking of trust, an adjustment one must make to the field of sports medicine is that the confidence that the athlete, coach, and parents have in the recommendations of the team physician correlates directly with the likelihood that these recommendations will be followed and not second-guessed. For the athlete, in most situations, the return to active participation in the shortest amount of time is the only focus. Blanket recommendations that focus on the illness and not the athlete's physiologic response to the illness will result in lost credibility, not only with the athlete, but often with the team and coaching staff as well. In its worst-case scenario this can lead to an "alternate" health care system, where an athlete or even an entire team will seek outside answers to medical issues. This problem can also occur when the team physician is limited in his or her availability to hold clinics or see athletes in the office setting. What is at issue here is more than a disjointed health care delivery system. Limited physician access compromises the critical role of the team physician in making return-to-play decisions. This does not imply that the team physician is the sole medical resource for the athlete, but when a consultant or second opinion is sought, the team physician should be the conduit for the interpretation of that decision and the ultimate arbitrator of when an athlete's condition will allow safe participation in athletics. Without the mandate to make return-to-play determination, a team physician becomes just another physician. Although administrative support for the team physician's decisions is essential, confidence in those decisions is only gained through trust. The cornerstone in developing this trust is accessibility.

BENEFITS OF ACCESSIBILITY

The team physician who is truly accessible rather than simply being seen on the sidelines once a week needs to be considered a highly valued member of the athletic health care team. Many benefits of this have been discussed earlier in this article, including an increased awareness of the needs of the ill or injured athlete, improved communication among the physician and multiple parties, and the establishment of trust. Another benefit of having an accessible team physician is the provision for continuity of care for those athletes who have existing medical conditions that need constant monitoring or treatment as they participate in athletics. Athletes who have conditions such as diabetes, asthma, attention deficit hyperactivity disorder, eating disorders, and so on truly benefit from having a team physician who is available and accessible to their unique needs. From the perspective of the athletic trainer and athletic administrator, the benefit of an accessible team physician is that it fosters an environment that allows for the creation of a true sports medicine team rather than a fragmented approach to athletic health care.

SUMMARY

As the world of competitive athletics and sports medicine rapidly evolves, the role of the team physician needs to keep pace. More and more athletes and coaches have increased pressures to succeed and win, and a byproduct of this pressure has been the increased demands placed on sports medicine departments and team physicians. No longer is it acceptable to have a team physician simply show up and stand on the sidelines. There is an expectation of physician accessibility to be readily available to evaluate and treat the ill or injured athlete, to effectively communicate with multiple parties the plan of care for the athlete, and to determine the return-to-play criteria that allow for the quick and safe return of the ill or injured athlete. Successful sports medicine departments have achieved their level of success in large part because they benefit from the services of a competent and accessible team physician.

References

[1] American Board of Internal Medicine. Subspecialty policies for sports medicine. Available at: http://www.abim.org/cert/policies_aqsports.shtm. Accessed March 2007.

[2] Steiner ME, Quigley DB, Wang F, et al. Team physician consensus statement. Am J Sports Med 2000;28:440–2.

[3] Steiner ME, Quigley DB, Wang F, et al. Team physician in college athletics. Am J Sports Med 2005;30:1545–51.

[4] Guskiewicz KM, Bruce SL, Cantu RC, et al. National Athletic Trainers' Association position statement: management of sports-related concussion. J Athl Train 2004;39(3):280–97.

Clin Sports Med 26 (2007) 161–172

CLINICS IN SPORTS MEDICINE

EVIER
NDERS

Understanding the Politics of Being a Team Physician

Joel L. Boyd, MD

TRIA Orthopaedic Center, 8100 Northland Drive, Bloomington, MN 55431, USA

T he team physician landscape is littered with political land mines. In the high-stakes world of professional sports, the politics of each encounter and medical decision—from figuring out how to get hired, to setting up a communication chain of command, to treating visiting players, to fending off the media—must be identified, assessed, and resolved. Key information must be communicated according to the expectations and unique personalities of each owner, general manager (GM), coach, trainer, and athlete. The best team physicians manage relationships, competing agendas, and politically charged circumstances as adeptly as they wield a scalpel.

THE POLITICS OF LANDING THE JOB

The first political hurdle is simply finding out that there's a position open. You won't find a "Wanted: Team Physician" classified ad in the local paper. Back in the day, it wasn't uncommon for a team owner to hire his golfing buddy as team physician—one Washington Redskins team physician was a dentist! Fortunately, as more money entered professional sports, medical expertise eventually trumped cronyism.

The wisest owners dutifully delegated the task of selecting a team physician. Although savvy owners, GMs, and coaches may know what they want in a wide receiver, shooting guard, or left winger, they understandably don't have any idea of what to look for in an orthopedist or medical doctor. A short list of candidates is usually pieced together by networking with local medical and community leaders.

As an African-American physician, I didn't travel in the same circles as the movers and shakers of the Minnesota sports scene. Still, I was excited when the National Hockey League (NHL) awarded an expansion team franchise to Minnesota in June 1997. The puck wouldn't be dropping at the first Minnesota Wild home game for 3 years, so that bought me some time to strategize. I already had a good hockey resume. Not only was I a member of the NHL's

E-mail address: joel.boyd@tria.com

0278-5919/07/$ – see front matter
doi:10.1016/j.csm.2006.12.002 © 2007 Published by Elsevier Inc.
sportsmed.theclinics.com

Diversity Task Force, I was team physician of the national USA Hockey team (from 1996 to the present day), and served in the same capacity for the International Hockey League's Minnesota Moose (from 1994 until the league was dissolved in 1996). I was also the medical director for the Minnesota State High School League, as well as team physician for all of Augsburg College's sports programs.

As a team physician candidate for a major league sports franchise, however, I was still flying under the radar. So I turned to Dave Mona, founder of Weber Shandwick Minneapolis, the Midwest's largest public relations firm. Dave and I had become friends after I moved to Minneapolis from Cleveland in 1990. Dave knew I was qualified for the job, but that I needed to be at the right events so I could meet the right people. Dave worked his connections to get me an invite to *Minneapolis Star Tribune* columnist Sid Hartman's annual picnic. Quite the coup. Sid, who has a beautiful house on the St. Croix River right outside of Minneapolis, is a local legend. His collection of "close personal friends" includes everyone from Bobby Knight to George Steinbrenner. Anybody who's anybody in Minnesota sports attends Sid's annual shindig.

I attended a couple of Sid's picnics. He probably still doesn't have a clue who I am, but I did meet the local sports elite, including Wild chief executive officer Jac Sperling (now the team's vice chairman). I also attended every Wild-related public event—announcement of the team name, unveilings of the team logo and team sweater, ground breaking home-ice ceremony for Xcel Energy Center. I'd leave my practice in the middle of the day just to go shake some hands and establish a presence.

The politicking paid off. I was invited to interview with general manager Doug Risebrough and Sheldon Burns, the team's recently hired medical director, and made the short list of four candidates. That's when the "partner politics" came into play—I was shocked to discover that David Fischer, my partner at TRIA Orthopaedic Center, was one of the final four. Not only had he encouraged me to go after the Wild opportunity—I believe his exact words were, "You've been here 10 years and it's time for you to have a team"—he was already team physician for both the Minnesota Vikings and Minnesota Timberwolves. Although David had little hockey experience, he told me that a member of the Wild brain trust, impressed with his team physician credentials, had recommended that the team also interview him. Fortunately, the tension between us dissolved when the Wild selected me. I suspect that David felt like the older brother who knew that his younger sibling would eventually start tugging away at what he had worked so hard to achieve. No matter how proud he is of his little brother, it's hard to let go.

Although most pro teams diligently seek out skilled physicians, a disturbing trend is gaining traction. More than twenty professional football, basketball, baseball, and hockey teams have awarded medical service provider contracts to the highest bidder. Some teams have reportedly collected up to $2 million from a mix of hospital systems, physician groups, and other health care organizations for the right to serve as official team "sponsors."

Granted, the medical provider will benefit from advertising exposure, community awareness, and the prestige that comes with being associated with the beloved home town team. Patient traffic is bound to increase. When Johnny falls and hurts himself, his parents will think, "If these guys are good enough to take care of the St. Louis Cardinals, they're good enough to take care of my kid."

Selecting medical service personnel based on financial factors raises ethical concerns, however. Many qualified physicians refuse to enter a bidding war as a matter of principle. Most important, when medical contracts are viewed as marketing agreements, players can rightfully question if they're receiving the best medical care, and where the physician's loyalty lies.

A team physician who has purchased the relationship may be more likely to expect exclusive access to injured players. Given that his qualifications have already been called into question, the physician may feel that his reputation is tarnished when a player seeks outside medical attention. Indeed, what message does that send to the rest of the team? To protect its financial interests, team ownership may be more likely to intervene on behalf of the team physician. The issue is especially sensitive because players, often at the urging of their agents, routinely consult with other medical providers.

Bottom line? Although selling the right to provide medical services may not compromise the quality of the medical care provided, it does open up a Pandora's box of potential abuse.

THE POLITICS OF STAKEHOLDER INTERACTION

Good team physicians are excellent communicators. They establish a clear chain of command and precise protocols, and expertly control and direct the flow of information. Without high-caliber communication skills, a team physician has no hope of managing the conflicting agendas of management, coaches, athletes, and the media.

The first order of business is to reach an understanding with the other team medical providers and athletic trainer regarding who speaks to the various stakeholders and under what conditions. The certified athletic trainer is often the first line of communication with team management and players, simply because he's on the premises more often and can often handle what needs to be communicated.

For more serious issues, designate yourself or the other team physician as the go-to guy for all communications. It's crucial that the medical staff speak with one voice. That's a challenge because other medical service providers generally want to share their facts and medical opinions directly with the parties involved. You can't let that happen. Allowing the GM, coach, players, and other non-medical personnel to receive reports from—and even arrange appointments with—multiple medical sources can be overwhelming and confusing. If you're the communication point man, and a player has a toothache, you need to be the one to set up the dental appointment. When the dentist reports back with his findings, it's you who should relay that information to the appropriate team personnel.

If you don't control the flow of information, you may find yourself out of the loop, which may affect your medical decisions going forward. Let's say a general surgeon calls the coach directly. Later, you come to practice and the coach tells you that the player is scheduled for surgery tomorrow. That makes you look foolish and uninformed. You should be telling such things to the coach, not the other way around.

Although creating medical protocols is the team physician's responsibility, it's essential to collaborate with team management and team medical personnel to make sure everyone's needs are being met. Preseason protocols, for instance, must address how players will be examined and evaluated to ensure that they're ready for the rigors of training camp and the upcoming season. What will player physicals include and who will perform them? Besides the standard orthopedic and medical examinations, should they be evaluated by a dentist? An ophthalmologist?

In the wake of a handful of tragic incidents involving star athletes, some physicians are advocating that every player should receive an echocardiogram. They point to the untimely death of Sergei Zholtok, a center for the NHL's Nashville Predators, who was diagnosed as having an irregular heartbeat in 2003 and died during a championship game in Belarus in November 2004. Detecting cardiac abnormalities, however, may generate serious political fallout. If you recommend that an athlete hang up his spikes as a medical precaution, you'll likely ignite a fiery debate and be challenged by the athlete as well as his team. If the team backs you, the player may retain an attorney and claim that his future earnings have been jeopardized. When large sums of money are at stake, long-term health often drops a notch on the priority scale.

The inevitability of injuries also demands airtight protocols. How will the injury get treated, rehabilitated, and resolved? Injuries will be either a musculoskeletal problem or a medical problem. As an orthopedic surgeon, musculoskeletal issues are right in my wheelhouse. The team's medical doctor will probably be consulted first if a player has a concussion, viral illness, or any number of other ailments.

The makeup and depth of a local team's medical staff vary tremendously depending on the sport, the league, and the market. Most teams have a head athletic trainer, an orthopedic surgeon, and a medical physician (an internist, general practitioner, or family practice doctor) who has an interest in sports medicine. At least one of these two team doctors is in attendance at every home game. (You'll also likely find a dentist at hockey games). Typically, because leagues want to deal with one medical representative per team, either the orthopedic surgeon or medical doctor is designated as the team's medical director.

The next tier of service providers may include a number of physicians of different subspecialties who don't necessarily attend games but are just a phone call away. The roster might consist of a team dentist, a team plastic surgeon, a team neurologist—pretty much every subspecialty you can imagine. Football is a notable exception in that all medical personnel typically travel to road games, and there may be as many as two doctors for each specialty—two orthopedists, two internists—because of the violent nature of the game.

Each group of stakeholders presents different challenges, as outlined below.

The Certified Athletic Trainer

The team physician needs to develop a friendly, yet mentor relationship with the head athletic trainer. During the season, I talk to the Minnesota Wild certified athletic trainer every day, and the Minnesota Lynx certified athletic trainer almost every day. In fact, I probably talk to them as much as I talk to my own family members!

One of the biggest mistakes a team physician can make is not giving the certified athletic trainer free rein. Except for extreme circumstances, the athletic trainer should be allowed to be the first on the scene to assess the situation and treat the injured player. The athletic trainer will then determine if the physician needs to venture out on the court, field, or ice. This builds the athletic trainer's confidence and lets the players know that he's qualified to take care of their medical needs. If the physician always rushes out at the first sign of trouble, the unspoken message is, "The athletic trainer isn't competent enough to be trusted." Bruising the athletic trainer's ego and undermining his authority in that way will likely damage the physician-athletic trainer relationship. There may also be more serious consequences. Remember, team physicians don't travel to away games except in football; not allowing the certified athletic trainer to be the first responder at home games may lead to a lack of self-assurance and experience, which in turn may lead to sub-par medical care on the road.

The Coach

I follow a simple rule: doctors should doctor, and coaches should coach. It may have been a plus that I knew very little about hockey before joining the Minnesota Wild. I enjoy the game but I can't even skate, so head coach Jacques Lemaire didn't have to worry about me trying to draw up any plays.

Although there's no master blueprint for dealing with coaches, they all have the same goal: they want their players to play. You have to figure out what information the coach wants and needs, and how to deliver that information. Some coaches I've worked with want to know every last detail of an injury or illness, whereas others just want to know when the player will be ready to suit up again. Some coaches want the certified athletic trainer to fill them in, whereas others won't settle for less than a full report from the team physician. Some coaches will be buddy-buddy with you, whereas others barely acknowledge your existence. Jacques Lemaire, for instance, rarely spoke to me. He'd listen to medical reports and only talk to me when necessary.

A coach's needs vary depending on the sport. If a Minnesota Vikings player is hurt on Sunday, head coach Brad Childress' primary concern will be whether he'll be ready to play the following Sunday; if not, the coaches will need to prepare another player to fill the position. Similarly, the Minnesota Timberwolves will need to give a bench player more practice time when a starter goes down. Hockey is a bit different. If a Minnesota Wild player goes down on Sunday and there's a game on Wednesday, the team will likely need to sign a free agent or call up a player from the Houston Aero's, the club's farm team. Either option is expensive. Contractual factors—is the free agent unrestricted?—also come into play. Granted, player contracts are not a physician's core competency, but because they influence the coach's personnel decisions, you should at least be familiar with the basics.

Although coaches and physicians share a common goal—keeping players healthy—there may be times when the team physician's agenda is diametrically opposed to the coach's. Take the time Minnesota Wild defenseman Brad Bombardier fractured his ankle in 2004. He had suffered the same injury in the past, which is always a concern, but from an orthopedic standpoint it was a classic, straightforward fracture. Eight weeks later, he started skating again. The team athletic trainer's injury reports were consistently positive.

Brad's attitude, however, didn't match up with the glowing medical reports. On game days, he would come in the locker room between periods with a hangdog look. I'd ask him what was wrong and he'd say, "I don't know, doc. I just don't have that push-off like I used to have." I'd take a radiograph and everything would look just fine. At practice the next day, the certified athletic trainer would tell me that Brad looked great, that he was "flying out there on the ice." It was a real head scratcher, until one day when the athletic trainer saw Brad talking to Jacques. When the conversation ended, the athletic trainer approached Brad and asked him what the coach had told him. "Jacques said I'm getting better but I just don't have that jump yet," Brad said.

Finally, I figured out what Jacques was up to. The defenseman who had been called up to replace Brad had been playing well. If Brad was activated, his replacement would have to be returned to the minors. But the team was winning, and Jacques didn't want to mess with the on-ice chemistry, so he figured he'd get a few more good games out of the replacement before taking Brad off of injured reserve. I had been looking at the situation strictly from a medical point of view, and understandably wondering why Brad wasn't getting better. As a team physician, you have to understand the game that coaches play with moving players around. It's a game within a game.

Visiting Teams

As a team physician, you're not a coach, you're not a player, you're not on staff. You represent the team, but you're basically alone on an island, governed by who needs medical care—no matter which team they play for. You need to view every player on every team as a unique individual patient. If a serious injury occurs to a visiting player, consult with the player's own physician and certified athletic trainer if you're concerned about how aggressively you should treat him. We take pride at the Minnesota Wild in knowing that opposing players who come to Xcel Energy Center receive excellent medical care. In fact, if a Dallas Stars player is injured in a Friday game, and the Stars have a weekend game with the Wild, Stars certified athletic trainer Dave Surprenant (who held a similar position with the Minnesota North Stars before they moved to Dallas in 1993) will often call ahead to ask us to examine and treat the player when the team arrives in Minnesota.

The General Manager

The GM's role fluctuates from team to team and sport to sport. I've been hired with a handshake by some GMs and never even met others. Many GMs stay out of the loop on medical issues, whereas others are intimately involved with protocols that spell out how injuries are reported and who they're reported to. Football GMs are minimally involved, basketball GMs a bit more so. Baseball GMs are moderately involved, and hockey GMs are very active.

The GM and the coach typically put their heads together to decide what the time requirements will be for the team physician position. Do they expect you to come to practice once or twice a week? Do they expect to see you only on game days? Do they want you there before the games to evaluate players? What about after the games? It's your job to find out the answers to all these questions.

The Media

Five words can make any team physician's job easier: don't talk to the media. If you must do so, lay out the facts, then yield the floor to the team spokesperson. Even then, the politics can get a bit dicey, because teams often don't want other teams to know who's hurt and to what extent. They may only want you to acknowledge that a player has an upper body or a lower body injury. Withholding health-related details can provide a competitive edge—loose lips sink championships. Your first day on the job is not too soon to find out your team's policy on releasing medical information.

Remember, the player is a patient, so all the laws and rules governing the doctor-patient relationship apply. Technically, without verbal consent from the player, you have no business talking about his injury with anyone else. That said, many teams are cavalier about the consent issue because players typically sign a waiver at the beginning of the season that effectively grants permission to team representatives to release factual medical information. Still, discretion is the better part of media relations. Even with a waiver, if a player gets diagnosed as having non-Hodgkin's lymphoma, I can get sued for disclosing that. When in doubt, turn toward the microphone or look into the camera, pause for dramatic effect, then speak the two words that every reporter dreads: "no comment."

Of course, when a star player is injured, your cell phone will ring incessantly. When Minnesota Twins catcher Joe Mauer tore his meniscus, one newspaper reporter left multiple voicemails. Finally, I returned his call and said that I couldn't talk to him about Joe's injury. He said, "Well, can you talk about meniscus injuries in general"? "Sure," I said, "I do that every day with patients." He went away satisfied because he had something to write for the next day's edition.

THE POLITICS OF MALPRACTICE INSURANCE

When Minnesota Vikings offensive lineman Korey Stringer succumbed to heat stroke in August 2001 after practicing in stifling humidity and temperatures over 90°, the NFL expanded its safety policies to include safeguards such as greater water and shade requirements, lighter uniform colors, and mandatory presence of a team physician at all practice sessions.

Stringer's death also had huge financial and medical implications for all US sports teams that travel to games against our neighbor to the north. Fearing substantial financial judgments, Canadian insurance companies dropped malpractice insurance for physicians who work with professional teams. That means that when the Minnesota Wild visit Montreal or Quebec or any other Canadian NHL city, the opposing team's medical staff can no longer treat our players at the rink—they have to be taken directly to a hospital.

Canada's abrupt withdrawal of malpractice insurance coverage raises significant legal, financial, political, and ethical concerns. Could it be challenged in court? Sure, but nobody has yet been willing to bankroll the effort. Before Canada revamped its rules, the team physician's malpractice insurance was covered under his professional practice; now it's an added expense. My guess is that it's only a matter of time before this excessive caution extends to collegiate teams. Sooner or later, an injured star athlete is going to claim that the college's doctor misdiagnosed or mistreated him, and will sue to be compensated for lost earning potential.

THE POLITICS OF INTERNATIONAL COMPETITION

Although local sports teams can typically draw from multiple medical resources for a variety of subspecialty care, the United States Olympic Committee (USOC) expects their team physicians to handle both musculoskeletal and medical issues.

As team physician for USA Basketball and USA Hockey, I was the only medical provider besides the certified athletic trainer to travel with the teams to non-Olympic contests. On a trip to Puerto Rico in 1997, my biggest challenge was treating one of the basketball coach's sons, who suffered a corneal abrasion from a body surfing face-plant. At the USA World Championships in Switzerland in 1998, I rushed to the hotel room of David Poile, the hockey team's GM, after he came down with food poisoning. On the same trip, I tended to a player's wife whose belly button became infected from a recent piercing. At the 1998 Winter Olympics in Nagano, Japan, TV sportscaster Mark Rosen caught a cold, and I was charged with tracking down some cough medicine for him. After a few international trips, I felt more like a general practitioner than an orthopedic surgeon.

The Olympics take place on a world stage, so it's not surprising that joining the US Olympic hockey team in the spring of 1997 led to my greatest political predicament. The team's GM was not happy that Ray Barile of the St. Louis Blues and I were picked as athletic trainer and team physician respectively. He wanted the doctor and certified athletic trainer from the World Cup team on the Olympic roster.

There were three good reasons why that wasn't going to happen. First, the World Cup is overseen by USA Hockey, whereas the Olympics are overseen by the USOC, so it wasn't the GM's call. Second, the USOC rigorously trains its medical providers to follow specific protocols to ensure that they can handle virtually any medical emergency, not just situations that fall within their specialty. Third, the USOC accredits its medical providers, and the physician and athletic trainer the GM was lobbying for weren't licensed to practice medicine in Japan.

Nonetheless, the GM remained adamant that his guys were going, not us. He instructed USA Hockey, which was still the governing body under the USOC umbrella, not to release our names to the media. Ten months later, the situation came to a head. USA Hockey arranged a meeting with the Olympics team medical staff during the 1998 NHL All-Star game festivities in Vancouver. The Olympics opening ceremony was less than 3 weeks away. Ray and I sat alone on one side of a huge conference table. Across from us sat the GM and the four-person medical staff he'd selected. As soon as the USA Hockey representative thanked everyone for coming, the GM announced that the meeting was a waste of time, and that we should cut to the chase. He pointed to Ray and me and said, "I don't want you or you to go." He then walked out. I thought, "Wow, now that was a fast meeting."

The USA Hockey rep followed the GM out and persuaded him to return. When we were all settled back in, I said to the GM, "I can understand why you're passionate about wanting your guys to go. I happen to know them, and there's no question that they're good at what they do. I want you to understand, however, that you and I haven't met, you don't know my qualifications, and besides, there are some things your people won't be able to do. First and foremost, they will not have a license to practice in Japan."

Ultimately, the USOC gave the GM permission to bring his own people, with the understanding that only Ray and I could treat the players. Privately, however, the GM made it clear to Ray and me that he didn't want us to even talk to the players, much less touch them. (In fact, he banned us from the team plane; we had to travel to Japan with other USOC staff on a separate flight.) Fortunately, the players understood the situation and came to us for treatment. When Brett Hull fractured a finger, I radiographed and injected it, and called his team physician back in the states to coordinate subsequent treatment. Those were the types of USOC protocols that the GM's handpicked physicians were unable to initiate without USOC accreditation.

THE POLITICS OF TREATING STAR PLAYERS

I scoped Minnesota Twins pitcher Carlos Silva's knee after he tore his meniscus near the end of the 2005 season. His knee felt fine during the first few months of the 2006 campaign—until it began swelling in July, which made it more difficult for him to keep his pitches down. The team was considering placing Silva on the 15-day disabled list, so John Steubs, the Twins' head club physician, sent Silva to my office for a Friday afternoon examination. He was scheduled to pitch against the White Sox on Sunday. The knee looked fine. I told Carlos, "I'll see you on Sunday. I'll be watching you." He laughed and left. I called John and said that Silva's knee would probably swell a bit after he pitched but that the athletic trainers should be able to calm it down in the 5 days before his next start, and that Silva would probably be good to go for the rest of the season.

Sunday turned out to be a beautiful July afternoon, so I gathered my charts, sat on my porch, and turned on the Twins game. Carlos walked the first man up while the announcers solemnly discussed his knee problems. The second batter drilled a laser into the upper deck in right field. My jaw dropped. I'd never seen a guy hit a ball that hard, that far. All I could think was, "Who was the idiot who said Silva could pitch?" I wondered if there was a good movie on—I couldn't bear to watch anymore. I could almost hear my phone ringing and Twins GM Terry Ryan asking me, "You sure he can play?" Thankfully, Silva settled down and gave the Twins six good innings, and his knee has held up just fine.

Joe Mauer's knee injury was a political free-for-all. It wasn't surprising: the Twins' young phenom catcher was the majors' top overall draft pick and a can't-miss prospect. In April 2004, in just his second major league game, Mauer injured his knee on a sliding attempt to catch a foul ball. By chance, Joe's cousin is married to an orthopedic surgeon who knew me and recommended to Joe that he see me, so the day after the injury, John Steubs and Joe were at my office. Sure enough, an MRI revealed a meniscus tear. The question was whether to remove the meniscus or repair it. It wasn't a simple decision. The MRI revealed a dislocated fragment, and the tear appeared to be a new tear on top of an old tear, so repairing it could be problematic. John and I agreed that the meniscus should be removed, which would keep Joe out of action for 6 to 8 weeks. (If the meniscus had been repairable, Joe would have been sidelined 3 to 6 months. In such cases, there's often a conflict between short-term and long-term goals.) I performed the operation, and 6 weeks later, Joe was swinging a hot bat for the Rochester Red Wings, the Twins' Triple-A farm club. Two more weeks and he was back in the majors.

Unfortunately, that wasn't the end of Joe's struggles. A month later, his knee was painful and swollen. He had played 5 days in a row, which would be a strain for a catcher who had healthy knees. I told John to take Joe off his anti-inflammatory medications so we could get the knee settled down and make sure the medications weren't masking any swelling or irritation. Another MRI showed a bone change inside his joint and increased inflammation. I recommended that Joe sit out, perhaps for the remainder of the season, to prevent further damage.

The Twins were in a quandary. To their credit, they had Joe's best interest at heart, yet they needed him on the field. Terry Ryan is a man of great character and unquestionable integrity, so I had no problem when he gave me a call to discuss his options. "Doc," he said, "we believe in you, we know you're doing the right thing, but Joe's family wants to get another opinion about his knee."

Joe's family wanted him to see an older, well-known orthopedic surgeon out West. On the surface, it made perfect sense to seek his opinion, but I told Terry that this doctor would probably want to perform surgery to address the findings of the second MRI. Although these findings were of concern, I didn't think surgery was warranted. Sure enough, Terry called me back after Joe had flown out West to confirm that the doctor had indeed recommended surgery. I told Terry that we had nothing to lose by sitting Joe down for 6 weeks to see if the knee calmed down. After all, if this new doctor operated on Joe, he'd be lost for the season, but by not operating, there was a good chance that Joe could return to the field that year or next without an operation. Terry agreed, and asked me to call the doctor in the hope of achieving consensus.

After leaving two or three voicemails, the doctor returned my call. We agreed that Joe was awfully young to be exhibiting the changes that showed up on the MRI, and that his knee was still relatively strong and healthy. I asked the doctor if there was any reason why the operation should be done now rather than wait 6 weeks in the hope that the knee would stabilize. The doctor agreed that waiting was the best option. Next thing I know, I'm on the phone again with Terry Ryan. Turns out that right after talking to me, the doctor told Joe's agent that Joe should have the surgery as soon as possible. Joe's agent tells Joe's family, who tells Terry Ryan, who calls me. Terry said, "Joel, I've got a real dilemma here. I've got one guy who's telling me that we should wait to see what happens and another guy who says we should operate. I think I'm going to get a third opinion. What do you think"? I encouraged Terry to do just that.

Terry ended up contacting Dr. John Bergfeld, one of my mentors at Cleveland Clinic. Having trained under him, I knew that Dr. Bergfeld would concur that it'd be best for Joe to wait 6 weeks instead of immediately going under the knife. I even told Terry that I'd help facilitate Joe's meeting with Dr. Bergfeld, which I did. After examining Joe, Dr. Bergfeld echoed my sentiment that it was rare for Joe's MRI changes to occur in someone his age. He said there was something odd going on and that it'd be best to wait to see if the knee calmed down before taking any drastic measures. He recommended that Joe do a series of exercises, along with bracing and other modalities. Dr. Bergfeld then called the doctor out West and told him what he had just recommended for Joe. Fortunately, Joe went with Dr. Bergfeld's recommendation.

When a high-profile player like Joe Mauer is injured, the media are relentless. The "Joe Watch" was a daily newspaper event. Granted, the baseball beat writers knew nothing of my behind-the-scenes maneuvering, so they couldn't connect all the dots. I'd pick up a newspaper and read that I had operated on Joe and now he wasn't playing, so thank goodness he was following Dr. Bergfeld's training protocol now. Hello? The papers made it sound like I had botched things up when just the opposite was true. It was also amusing to see myself quoted in the press when I hadn't talked to any reporters. Apparently, Terry had told the reporters what I had told him and they included those second-hand quotes as if I had spoken directly to them.

Of course, today's politics becomes yesterday's news awfully fast. Joe's knee was all that mattered. Joe didn't return that season, which was a smart move.

He rehabilitated his knee over the winter, had a solid 2005, and as I write this, is leading the major leagues in hitting in September 2006. His knee is strong as it can be and his future looks bright.

SUMMARY: THE TWELVE-STEP "PHYSICIANS AND POLITICS" PROGRAM

The more prepared and professional you are, the fewer political land mines you'll trip. Avoid needless and embarrassing gaffes by adhering to these twelve tips:

1) Pay your dues. Start working with local sports teams to gain experience.
2) Create visibility. Make yourself known to team decision-makers.
3) Communicate clearly. Professional communication training is a plus.
4) Build relationships. Sports is like life: it's all about relationships.
5) Create protocols. A disorganized doctor is an ineffective doctor.
6) Establish a chain of command. Let others know who to talk to and when.
7) Direct the flow of information. A team needs to speak with one voice.
8) Clarify expectations. Determine the needs and wants of each stakeholder.
9) Give your certified athletic trainer free rein. It'll help build confidence and expertise.
10) Let the coaches coach. Don't stick your nose where it doesn't belong.
11) View each player as an individual. That goes for visiting players, too.
12) Be wary of the media. If you must talk to them, stick to the facts.

Follow these guidelines, and your tour of duty as team physician will be smoother and more gratifying. Serving as team physician for a number of different sports, both professional and amateur, has been enormously rewarding. It feels good to give back to the community in this way while also making a positive impact on your favorite local teams. Best of luck to you. I hope that you enjoy the experience as much as I have.

Clin Sports Med 26 (2007) 173–179

CLINICS IN SPORTS MEDICINE

SEVIER
UNDERS

Building a Sports Medicine Team

Freddie H. Fu, MD, HDSc*, Fotios Paul Tjoumakaris, MD,
Anthony Buoncristiani, MD

Department of Orthopaedic Surgery, Center For Sports Medicine, 3200 South Water Street,
Pittsburgh, PA 15203, USA

B uilding a winning sports medicine team is equally as important to the success of an athletic organization as fielding talented athletes. Acquisition of highly qualified, motivated, and hard-working individuals is essential in providing high quality and efficient health care to the athlete. Maintaining open paths of communication between all members of the team is the biggest key to success and an optimal way to avoid confusion and pitfalls.

There have been a growing number of participants in high school and collegiate athletics in recent years, placing ever-increasing demands on the sports medicine team. With tremendous advances in athletic medicine and the specialization of medical care increasing in the United States, a wide array of specialists are now deemed necessary to care for athletes. Questions arise as to who should serve as part of the sports medicine team, which care provider should serve as the coordinator, what are the defined roles of each member, and how can a coordinated approach be maintained to best care for the athlete? The answers to all of these questions have been hotly debated over the years [1]; however, some agreement exists as to the importance of each member to create a coordinated and comprehensive approach to medical coverage, providing optimal care for the athlete [1].

This article outlines the importance of each member of the sports medicine team and provides a guideline for sports medicine physicians on how to assemble the optimal team of specialists in order to provide the best medical care for the athlete. Defining which members warrant inclusion and how care is administered are discussed.

OBJECTIVES OF THE SPORTS MEDICINE TEAM

Before any process of assembling the proper players for the team can begin, a basic paradigm or mission statement is critical to defining the objectives of the sports medicine team. This technique is often used in corporations to clearly identify the objectives of the corporation, the consumers that it serves,

*Corresponding author. Center for Sports Medicine, University of Pittsburgh Medical Center, 3200 S. Water St., Pittsburgh, PA 15203. E-mail address: ffu@upmc.edu (F.H. Fu).

0278-5919/07/$ – see front matter
doi:10.1016/j.csm.2006.12.003
© 2007 Published by Elsevier Inc.

and the employees who achieve its end [2]. The same basic paradigm can be applied to the sports medicine team. The health team must identify the objectives that it must achieve, provide a quality product to the athlete, and provide the providers with a sense of contribution. In the year 2000, the team physicians' consensus statement was outlined from collaboration among six sports medicine and medical societies [3]. Within this statement lies an excellent outline for the objectives of the sports medicine team:

- Coordinate pre-participation screening, evaluation, and examination.
- Manage injuries on the field.
- Provide for medical management of injury and illness.
- Coordinate rehabilitation and return to participation.
- Provide for proper preparation for safe return to participation after an illness or injury.
- Integrate medical expertise with other health care providers, including medical specialists, athletic trainers, and allied health professionals.
- Provide for appropriate education and counseling regarding nutrition, strength and conditioning, ergogenic aids, substance abuse, and other medical problems that could affect the athlete.
- Provide for proper documentation and record keeping.

This paradigm of care, in effect, is our mission statement. When assembling the team, it is paramount to ensure that all aspects of this mission are achieved through the use of our players in an appropriate fashion. The following is an example of a clear and inclusive mission statement from the James Madison University Sports Medicine Team that sets objectives and outlines a multidisciplinary approach to the care of the athlete: "The Department of Sports Medicine aspires to be a leader in providing quality healthcare services to all student-athletes. A team of multi-skilled professionals, utilizing current research, educational knowledge, and state-of-the-art equipment and technology, strives to provide a comprehensive and progressive approach to assuring the holistic well being of each student-athlete."

WHO MAKES THE CUT?

The first decision that must be made in the overall assembly of our team is to identify which care providers are essential players and which can be used more in an ancillary capacity. Although it may at first glance seem best to apply an all-inclusive approach to this question, requesting the help of a multitude of providers from various disciplines, a more careful analysis of this question shows that a "less is more" doctrine may provide for clearer communication, less confusion for the athlete and personnel, and more efficient delivery of health care.

The "gatekeeper" of the sports medicine team and the provider on the "front lines" of this process is the certified athletic trainer. Not only is this person the most likely first contact for the athlete with a medical concern, this individual is often intimately involved with the athlete on a personal level, and should an injury warrant treatment, the certified athletic trainer is often the provider ad-ministering the treatment program. Most athletic injuries occur during practice, not during the game when physician supervision is often present. The certified athletic trainer is perfectly suited to address injuries in this setting. In addition, data from high schools suggests that one in five high school athletes will sustain an athletic injury during their careers [4]. This large volume of injuries war-rants a front line manager who can diagnose, examine, triage, refer, and treat patients appropriately.

The sports medicine physician is the next critical player in the starting lineup. The sports medicine physician must meet certain criteria to qualify for this position:

- Have an MD or DO degree with an unrestricted license to practice medicine.
- Possess fundamental knowledge of providing emergency care for sporting events.
- Be trained in CPR; assistance with emergency medical services (EMS) for certain events may be warranted (eg, football).
- Have a working knowledge of trauma, musculoskeletal injury, and medical conditions affecting the athlete [3].

Additional desirable but not always possible requirements for the sports phy-sician are: specialty board certification, continuing education in sports medicine, fellowship training in sports medicine, significant practice contribution to the care of athletes, and membership and participation in a sports medicine society.

Vital players of the team are the coach and coaching staff of the injured ath-lete—from the head and assistant coaches to the strength and conditioning coach for the team. A strong working relationship with open communication is necessary between the medical staff and the coaches to optimize care for the athlete. It should be clear to all parties that they share a common objective: the safe return to play of the injured athlete. Several studies have documented the ethical dilemma inherent in this relationship between medical personnel and coaching/ownership staff; however, with open communication and clear understanding of this fundamental objective, this dilemma can be minimized [5]. The strength and conditioning coach can be employed as part of the treatment program, allowing the athlete to continue to feel part of the team during a long rehabilitation process.

In addition to the certified athletic trainers, physician, and coaching staff, it is helpful to view the athletes' parents (for collegiate and high school athletics) as parts of the team as well. These emotional supporters of the athlete are crucial to the successful treatment of injured players. The entire emotional support net-work from teammates, family, and friends cannot be underestimated. Shared experiences and encouragement during rehabilitation provide much needed support, and are often as valuable as the medical treatment itself.

This basic setup of the sports medicine team is an adequate beginning to car-ing for the injured athlete; however, it is only the beginning. This foundation is just that, a place to start. Several more providers are necessary for the comprehensive care of the athlete. The sports medicine physician should have access to an array of medical and ancillary providers, all adept at treating injured athletes. This access should be expedient, providing competent and quick decision-making. If the physician is a primary care sports medicine provider, a close working relationship with an orthopedic surgeon (preferably trained in sports medicine) is paramount. The reverse is true if the primary medical provider is an orthopedic surgeon. The physician should have quick access to specialists in the fields of hand surgery, foot and ankle surgery, neurosurgery/neurology, ophthalmology, internal medicine, general surgery, dentistry, and radiology. Ancillary providers such as sports specific physical therapists, nutritionists, and sports psychologists round out the medical team, providing the most comprehensive care in the best of scenarios. Game coverage by EMS is also important to stabilize critically injured athletes on the field of play. Fellows, residents, and athletic training students undergoing training in sports medicine often play an integral role in facilitating prompt care when access to the senior staff is difficult.

Often times the athletic director is involved in coordinating and organizing the team in coordination with a designated team physician and athletic trainer. The budget allocated to the care of athletes will ultimately determine which providers are included or excluded from participation.

COORDINATION OF CARE

As mentioned previously, there has been significant debate in the medical community regarding who is best suited to be the sports medicine director of the medical team. Rather than contribute to this debate, the authors find it best to give parameters by which to judge a suitable candidate. First and foremost, it must be recognized that the true "coordinator" of care for athletes is the certified athletic trainer. This position requires an individual who is not only skilled in the ability to diagnose and treat musculoskeletal conditions, but who possesses excellent organizational and communication skills. The certified athletic trainer is responsible for coordinating pre-participation examinations, training room evaluations, referrals to the physician, and accurate record keeping for the athlete's medical record, including health care insurance coverage and payment. A study on the perception of certified athletic trainers by student athletes demonstrated that, overall, student athletes had a very good perception of their certified athletic trainers [6]. This perception places the certified athletic trainer in a key role as athlete advocate and practitioner. As if this task weren't daunting enough, the certified athletic trainer often serves as the liaison between the coaches and physicians and between athletes and their parents, which requires tremendous interpersonal and communication skills.

The overall director of medical care should be an individual who possesses many of the same qualities as the certified athletic trainer. At the very core of these qualities is a significant level of competence in the field of musculoskeletal medicine. A recent study performed on intercollegiate athletes at a Division I University demonstrated that 73% of all training room visits by athletes were for a musculoskeletal complaint [7]. The visits for musculoskeletal injuries among athletes were much more likely to require repeat evaluation, whereas visits for common medical diagnoses (respiratory tract infection and so forth) were not. In addition, 4% of all musculoskeletal injuries ultimately required some form of surgical intervention. For this reason, it is critical that the medical director of the sports medicine team be an individual who is trained in musculoskeletal medicine. The roles of the director include

- Establish and define the relationships of all parties.
- Educate athletes, parents, coaches, administrators and other parties of concern regarding the athletes.
- Develop a chain of command.
- Plan and train for emergencies during games and practice.
- Address equipment and supply issues.
- Provide for proper event coverage.
- Assess environmental concerns and playing conditions.
- Provide oversight for clinical policies and procedures, (concussion management, dehydration, and so forth) [3].

Several schools and professional teams may often request that this individual be a sports medicine-trained orthopedic surgeon, because decisions regarding surgical intervention are often made on a continual basis. This may be necessary at certain levels of competition; however, in some instances a well-trained primary care sports medicine specialist may be sufficient. The important point is that this individual must have open paths of communication and demonstrate superior leadership qualities.

AVOIDING PITFALLS, CONFUSION, AND CONFLICTS

When assembling the team, it is important that all parties recognize their roles in the chain of command to avoid confusion and overlap between the players. The sports medicine physician sets the tone and must clearly communicate to all parties what is expected of them. Having a written outline documenting the responsibilities of each individual can significantly reduce the amount of overlap between different providers, and can help to avoid conflicts when they arise. An example of such a scenario may be that the internal medicine consultants relegate themselves to decision-making regarding non-musculoskeletal issues (asthma, heart conditions, and so forth), whereas the orthopedic consultants focus solely on that topic. Providers must be given a certain level of autonomy in the decision-making process in order to feel as if they are contributing to the overall care of the athletes. Confusion arises when several parties are rendering differing opinions on the care of the athlete and a clear rehabilitation program is not outlined. This could have an adverse impact, especially with respect to return-to-play expectations of athletes and coaches.

Primary care sports medicine specialists may have anticipated being an integral part of the musculoskeletal decision making process, only to find that they are being used in a capacity more suitable for a medical internist. Asking pertinent questions when being asked to be a member of the team can help avoid this potential conflict of objectives. In addition, orthopedic surgeons and their primary care colleagues may have differing views on the optimal management of some common nonoperative injuries. Meeting regularly to discuss these issues can help the team come to a protocol for the optimal delivery of health care in these instances. Having a well-qualified, certified athletic trainer cannot be underestimated in avoiding several conflicts. It should be clear to the certified athletic trainer which injuries warrant bumping up to the next level in the chain of command. The medical director may decide that nonoperative injuries (sprains, contusions, and so forth) be evaluated by members who do not perform surgery, and that more serious injuries should be evaluated by the surgeon. Whichever decision is made, a certain level of autonomy must be given to the treating individual when evaluating these patients and coordinating a treatment plan. The inclusion of specialists into the treatment algorithm should flow through the sports medicine director. The director should have clear communication with the specialists, whether they are being used to render treatment or a medical opinion. Obviously, the athlete has certain rights in this regard, but usually defers to the medical staff for the coordination of care.

All members of the team should meet regularly, both during the season and in the off-season, to discuss various issues that arise regarding conflicts, difficult cases requiring high level decision-making, and any overlap that may be hindering efficient delivery of care. Regularly scheduled training room sessions in which athletes are evaluated are an integral part of this efficient delivery. Staffing of these sessions is the responsibility of the director and the certified athletic trainer. The use of e-mail can serve as a useful adjunct, and can be used to determine if patients warrant radiographs or other diagnostic tests before being seen by the physician. E-mail also allows all members to discuss issues regularly, and is essential in keeping the lines of communication open. The physician and certified athletic trainer should meet with the coach on a regular basis to discuss all injuries and their responses to treatment. Parents should be introduced into the equation as quickly as possible, and having one spokesman in this regard is essential to avoid confusion and allay fears. Signed releases allowing the team to release information to parents for athletes over the age of 18 is required to involve family in the decision-making process.

ESTABLISHING A WINNING TEAM

The sports medicine team does not have the benefit of a lackluster season, nor can a "rebuilding" phase be accommodated. It is essential that all members of the team are on their "A" game at all times. Obviously, as members of the team work together longer and solidify strong working relationships, the team will only get stronger and more efficient. The key to success in this regard is to never surrender the strong foundation of availability, affability, and ability. All personnel should be available to the athlete and to each other for rendering of care. All parties should recognize that each has something to contribute and should respect the opinions of all stakeholders. All parties should also be qualified to render medical care in the highest capacity possible. Regular attendance at courses and continuing medical education is required to render the best treatment that science has to offer.

The component of trust among team members is important to create the optimal atmosphere for patient care. All members of the team should feel confident in their own ability as well as the coordinated ability of the staff to provide the most current and appropriate medical care. Attendance at conferences by all parties and cross-disciplinary education is essential to create this atmosphere. Certified athletic trainers should be offered opportunities to observe surgery on athletes, and physicians should be encouraged to attend athletic training conferences and symposia. In this fashion, all members of the team create an appropriate check-and-balance situation to ensure the highest degree of trust and confidence among stakeholders.

The essential component to sustaining a winning team is communication. The importance of this concept cannot be emphasized enough. As long as open lines of communication are continually maintained, all conflicts can be resolved and all shareholders can be accommodated. The old adage "There is no 'I' in team" is appropriate when caring for the athlete. Recognition of a coordinated approach to athletic care is imperative to sustain the best possible working relationship. Our focus as practitioners of health care should be on the patient as much as possible, with sound protocols in place that support our objectives of competent, efficient delivery of care. Laying a strong foundation from the beginning will pay dividends when game time approaches.

References

[1] Matheson G. Orthopaedics vs. primary care: time for a cease-fire [editorial]. Phys Sportsmed 2002;4–8.
[2] Covey SR. Universal mission statement. In: Covey SR. Principle centered leaderhip. New York: Free Press; 1990. p. 295–302.
[3] AOSSM. Team physician consensus statement. Am J Sports Med 2000;28:440–2.
[4] Lyznicki JM, Riggs JA, Champion HC. Certified athletic trainers in secondary schools: report of the council on scientific affairs. American Medical Association. J Athl Train 1999;34(3): 272–6.
[5] Tucker AM. Ethics and the professional team physician. Clin Sports Med 2004;2:227–41.
[6] Unruh S. Perceptions of athletic training services by collegiate student-athletes: a measurement of athlete satisfaction. J Athl Train 1998;33(4):347–50.
[7] Steiner ME, Quigley B, Wang F, et al. Team physicians in college athletics. Am J Sports Med 2005;33(10):1545–51.

Clin Sports Med 26 (2007) 181–185

CLINICS IN SPORTS MEDICINE

:VIER
NDERS

Establishing a New Practice as a Team Physician

J. Scott Quinby, MD

Sports Medicine Clinic of North Texas, 1015 North Carroll Avenue, Suite #2000, Dallas, TX 75204, USA

E stablishing a new practice, in and of itself, is extraordinary challenging. Trying to simultaneously establish oneself as a team physician can be particularly difficult. With persistence and motivation, the results can be very rewarding.

Unless medical school and residency leisure time were spent learning the principles of business, accounting, economics, and marketing, most of your education in these areas will come from your experiences the first few years in practice. Although these experiences sometimes present themselves during sports fellowship training, the vast majority of learning occurs when you have finally entered "the real world" of practice.

PRACTICE SETTING

Practice settings vary widely, and even if you are returning to your old familiar town, you are going to experience a side of it you have never recognized before. Unless you enter an academic institution where relationships have long been established, there will not be a department chairman or fellowship coordinator to take you under his wing.

A vast majority of those finishing fellowship training will be entering the private sector in a large metropolitan setting where competition can be fierce. The private setting can vary from joining a well-established group, with equally well-established referral patterns, to trying to fly solo where most would be inheriting a retiring surgeon's practice. Either way, you are the new kid on the block and will sometimes be met with skepticism. Establishing yourself as a team physician in this environment largely depends on word of mouth and a helpful hand from your new partners. One undisputed fact is that "beating the streets" is an essential component of success, as your competition will not be serving up the nearby school as a "welcome to practice" gift.

Joining a group that has existing relationships with multiple schools can be an opportunity to spend some time with experienced senior partners. Typically there are more than enough games that require coverage, and offering your

E-mail address: quinby2@hotmail.com

0278-5919/07/$ – see front matter
doi:10.1016/j.csm.2006.12.004
© 2007 Elsevier Inc. All rights reserved.

services to those teams typically underserved (eg, junior varsity basketball, women's sports) will be greatly appreciated. Just as having senior partners can be an opportunity for growth, the time they have spent developing their own practices can lead to possessive, and for that matter protective, attitudes toward "their" schools. Finding a balance so as to not upset the homeostasis is beneficial to relationship-building in the community.

Solo practice brings new challenges, but also new opportunities. The homeostasis of the community is more justifiably disrupted in this setup, because disruption may be required to build your practice. Also, being solo allows you to establish your own relationships without having to answer to the partners who are paying your salary. The solo setting would unquestionably require a general orthopedics approach for an extended period of time to be able to cover your overhead expenses.

An academic setting or multispecialty group or hospital may allow for greater referrals from within the group, but has its own drawbacks. Academic settings more typically involve a group of subspecialists and fewer general orthopedists, allowing for less competition for the same patient among partners. Building a professional referral base is quickly established because it is unlikely for a department or group to bring someone on who is not desperately needed. The resources of the institution also allow for more attractive options for athletic organizations for inexpensive "one-stop" shopping. The drawbacks are clearly less autonomy and still having to answer to a chairman or board of directors that may choose which direction you point your practice in.

One thing that must always be remembered is that most orthopedists consider themselves as "sports docs." Outside of orthopedics, the chiropractors, family practice sports specialists, and even the obstetrics/gynecology doctors are vying for taking care of the athletes. The bottom line is that even though you, as a sports fellowship-trained orthopedist, may be the most qualified for being the team physician, you don't look any different from the stands.

TEAM PHYSICIAN BENEFITS

The benefits of establishing oneself as a team physician are particularly significant for the surgeon just starting a practice. A common misconception is that as the official "team doc" you will be providing all orthopedic care for every athlete at that institution. Depending on the level of competition (ie, junior high, high school, club sport, collegiate, professional), many of the athletes already have an established relationship with an orthopedist. Many of the referrals that are part of your growing practice are actually teachers, administrators, school officials, and the parents of athletes. Becoming a family's team doc goes a long way when friends get together to talk about their ailments and your name comes up in the discussion. Providing good, friendly care in an expedited fashion is sometimes the only thing that separates you from the established community orthopedist.

Game coverage is almost invariably uncompensated, and is typically required in order for you to be the team's provider. Because increasing your liability is a realistic concern, the joy of being an integral part of the adrenaline-pumped athletic event is compensation enough. The fans are interested in who that is out on the field rendering care to their favorite player. This in turn generates more conversation (hopefully positive) and potentially future referrals. Time spent on the sidelines with the athletic trainer, coach, and athletic director also renders dividends because "curbside" consults are a regular half-time event. Finally, the visiting team's bench is frequently not covered by an orthopedist, presenting yet another opportunity to broaden your potential referral base.

When building a sports practice, doctor-shopping by athletes becomes the *Who's Who* of the athletic world. Taking care of a prestigious team renders you as a more qualified orthopedist in the eyes of the athlete. Why would that team or school be using Dr. So-and-So unless he was the best? The name of the surgeon who operated on the team quarterback who will take his team to a title is important information. Just as this can have very positive outcomes for practice development, the quarterback's future performance becomes a reflection of your ability as a surgeon, and could be detrimental. Just keep in mind that there are many Monday-morning quarterbacks out there, and that public opinion of the team doc can be dynamic.

COMMITMENTS AND RESPONSIBILITIES

Once the jockeying for position has secured a role as the official team physician, you are now at least committed to all of one team's home games. That commitment is typically the bare minimum, and can go to the extreme of attending all practices, daily training room, weekend games, traveling with the team, and attendance at team meetings—all this while trying to build an infant practice and be available for your other patients who require your attention. This also coincides with commitments made to your family, who have just moved to a new house and city and have already been taking lower priority than your practice.

Responsibilities largely include those to the athletic trainer, who is answering to the coach and athletic director. Lack of communication will make the athletic trainer's job much more difficult, and your status as the "go-to doc" guarded at best. The athletic trainer's impression of you as a physician will either help build your practice with frequent referrals or make the team physician job just an added time commitment.

Orthopedic care of athletes typically follows traumatic injury during play, and is not a scheduled event. This means that the team doc must be available, at least by phone, at all times. Being available at a family's or team's desperate time of need may not always coincide with your schedule, but will very clearly pay dividends. Extra hours and easy accessibility are important when fostering a relationship with a team. Personal sacrifice and time commitment are common among those working with a team in any capacity (ie, athletic trainers, coaches, juice crew, and so forth), and the same commitment on the part of the team physician is greatly appreciated.

NETWORKING

Marketing your new practice is an essential component of its growth. Specific time set aside from patient care and the business side of things must be dedicated to strategizing how to get patients in your clinic door. What better time to educate yourself on the market situation than while watching a sporting event?

Game coverage affords many opportunities to chat with the athletic trainer, coaches, parents, and referees. Some of the best market analysis comes from talking with the athletes who already have established relationships with another orthopedist. A knee brace can be a red flag and a good conversation starter that can lead to a potential future patient. Taking extra time to offer your expertise at no charge can leave a lasting impression. A chance to potentially alleviate a nagging knee injury may be just what the athlete needed but was afraid to ask for.

ADDITIONAL RESOURCES

Using all potential resources includes those provided by the hospital's marketing department, your practice's marketing person if it has one, manufacturer representatives, and anyone else that could potentially benefit from your getting busy. Because most collegiate and professional teams these days are contractually covered by hospital systems, your role as a sports specialist within that system provides for opportunity that would otherwise be out of reach. Developing relationships with your colleagues on staff at the hospital could create reciprocal referral patterns that quickly shunt patients into your office. This can also hold true for the physical therapists who are treating your patients. Because they depend on your business for their own survival, they can only benefit from your having greater numbers of potentially therapy-requiring patients.

LESSONS LEARNED

Entering a highly competitive marketplace and having to dedicate considerable time to establishing one's position in the sports community is not the expectation of most orthopedic residents. After the many years of hard work and developing the confidence of a qualified surgeon, the naïve opinion is that everything will fall into place and your staff will take care of the rest. The cruel reality is that you have only been given the tools to be a good surgeon and doctor, but remain particularly green to the business of orthopedics. Sure, there are friendly sources of information and guidance to provide some insight to your new world, but your quickly expanding experience becomes your greatest asset. Trial and error becomes the greatest opportunity for growth, despite attempts at previously conceived plans of infallible marketing techniques. The key is to learn from your own mistakes and those of your more experienced partners.

SUMMARY

The role of a team physician is an integral part of establishing a new practice. Regardless of the type of practice one enters, the team physician role provides an opportunity to establish an early referral base to build the foundation of a successful practice. Although this comes with great responsibility and significant time commitments, the joy of developing your practice doing what you enjoy most, sports medicine, makes these drawbacks less perceptible. Using all your potential resources and keeping your eye on the ball will simplify reaching the goal of having a happy, healthy, and rewarding career.

Clin Sports Med 26 (2007) 187–191

CLINICS IN SPORTS MEDICINE

Balancing Life as a Team Physician

Mary Lloyd Ireland, MD

Kentucky Sports Medicine, 601 Perimeter Drive, Suite 200, Lexington, KY 40517, USA

When I think of balancing acts, including my own, the first image that comes to mind is one of those old photographs depicting a circus artist slowly walking across a wire strung high above the center ring. The lights in the big tent are dimmed and the crowd stares up at the solitary figure, wondering if the worst could possibly happen while, of course, being simultaneously thrilled, because in the darkness below there is no net.

Invariably, these daring acts ended happily, with the circus barker proclaiming the performer's great courage, even as the clowns rushed into the center ring with their huge, grotesquely painted smiles and glittering eyes. If any of my friends should happen to be reading this, let me quickly make it clear that the remark about clowns was not intended to be a subtle reference to the man I married. He is not a clown. But he has certainly had a few, shall we say, entertaining moments. For example:

We were traveling together with friends in Kenya several years ago, touring game preserves, and I had brought along a basic medical kit in case there was a problem. When we arrived at a well-known resort called "Ol Malo," my husband pointed to a small crowd of Masai women and children congregated around the resort's entrance gates.

"Who are those folks?," he inquired of the resort owner.

"Well, those are just some locals who are looking for something to eat. The drought has been severe. Now, the men are away taking care of their cattle and goats, looking for water and food," the man replied.

My husband stared at the rather pathetic scene for a moment. "You know," he said, turning to the owner, "I can't help you with the drought, but my wife is an orthopedic surgeon and she's got a medical kit with her. I'm sure she'd be willing to help if any of those people back there have health problems."

Lesson number one is that it's tough to strangle someone sitting behind you in the back seat, but as the Range Rover hurried through the gate, the ranch owner turned to me with a smile and said, "Hey, that's really nice of you to offer. I'll keep that in mind."

Exactly 1 hour later, I was hustled aboard a private helicopter with my ridiculously inadequate medical kit and whizzed away to tend to a neighboring

E-mail address: ksm@kysportsmed.com

0278-5919/07/$ – see front matter
doi:10.1016/j.csm.2007.01.001
© 2007 Elsevier Inc. All rights reserved.
sportsmed.theclinics.com

rancher who, I was told, had just been gored by an elephant. My husband, of course, was sound asleep the whole time, taking his afternoon nap.

I washed out his wounds with what appeared to be an antiseptic solution. He had back pain. Fearing I might find a tusk wound in his back, I rolled him over. Skin intact and pain left flank—kidney contusion, I thought. He was biting his knife handle for pain control. I asked for assistance in opening the normal saline. A nearby Samburu warrior immediately whipped out his machete and whacked off the top of the saline bottle with one swipe. I politely said "Thank you."

Fortunately, this particular balancing act ended happily. I got the injured rancher stabilized; intravenous started, and cleaned out his wounds before he was transported by another helicopter to a hospital in Nairobi. I remember, as I rode back to the ranch, thinking about how unpredictable accidents are. And how alike they all are, too, as they lie in wait to spring at us from the shadows, confident that we will never see them coming. Best to be on your toes, then, your eyes wide open, and on your good days, trembling with anticipation.

MY PERSONAL TEN COMMANDMENTS

Balancing my job as a sports medicine doctor with my interests in research and training and the demands of my family and friends has been a great challenge, a kind of high wire act on a daily basis, occasionally with no net. But here they are: my personal "Ten Commandments" for maintaining your balance. A few may seem obvious, but don't be deceived. The easy sounding ones are often the most difficult to follow.

Do the Right Thing, Always, no Exceptions

A famous coach at the University of Kentucky, where I was once the team physician, confronted me about medical advice I had given to one of his players. The student had had an anterior cruciate ligament (ACL) reconstruction several years before and was unstable with a meniscus tear and early arthritis. He wanted to continue playing (don't they all) and put off the surgery to post season.

"Doc," he said, "if I hurt my knee again could it affect my pro career"?

"Yes," I replied. "More importantly, it could affect you. I am not sure you can play the rest of this season, much less in the pros. You will do harm to yourself if you play on an unstable knee and you may have pain in the future, even with everyday activity."

"I want to play now. I'm not worried about the future. Can I play this season"?

I told him. "No. Don't take a chance on a life-altering injury in hopes of playing this season or making it in the pros. Have the operation now."

When he heard about the advice I had given his player, the coach immediately hauled me into his office and, when I refused to change my tune, I was replaced as the team physician. So, even if it hurts you, even if it hurts the team and the coach, don't budge an inch when it comes to the welfare of the individual athlete. And no, I'm not going to mention the coach's name. There are too many coaches just like him who will not take their eyes off of winning and, when they submit to a "win-at-all-costs" method of coaching, they are not the team physician's, or the athlete's, friend.

It is Better to be an Advocate than Curse your Competition

This particular commandment is based loosely on an old proverb, "It is better to light a candle than curse the darkness."

The first fact of life most physicians must face is competition for patients, and this is especially true in the field of sports medicine, where the most gifted athletes are also local or even national celebrities. If you are a female in a medical specialty heavily dominated by men—intelligent, aggressive, successful men—you should become an advocate for issues that really mean something to you. Currently, only 2% of board-certified orthopedists are women, but more women in sports will inevitably mean more women in sports medicine in general and more women in orthopedics specifically. This is a good thing, for the profession as well as female athletes. Those of us blazing the trail for these future physicians should grab every opportunity to mentor and encourage young women to consider orthopedics as a female-friendly specialty.

Don't Demand Respect from Players and Coaches, Earn it

A number of people made a big deal out of the fact that I was the first woman in America to serve as team physician for a Division One team. But what really made me proud was the day I read a quote in the newspaper from a University of Kentucky football player who said, "We don't classify her as a woman or man—just like it doesn't matter if you're white or black. What matters is she knows what she is doing." I did know what I was doing, and the players could tell.

Loyalty is the Weakest of Human Values

I've never had a contract with any of the high school, college, or university sports programs I've worked with. That means I basically provided the service(ie, attending the games and practices, examining and treating the athletes on the field and in the training room) for free. I employed the athletic trainers and the school stipend was 30% of their salary. Over 10 years I donated (not tax deductible!) a lot of time and money. From this relationship, the practice grew, but insurance reimbursements fell. I was unable to "donate" these services. When another medical group bid on taking over my high school relationships, basically offering to pay the entire salary of all the school athletic trainers, the school board completely ignored my years of free service. One of the board members remarked during a hearing: "We should look at this just like we look at contracts for providing milk to the cafeteria." I did not even get a "thank you" for 10 years of service. If you lose a team or patient, get over it. There will be other opportunities. Focus on what you can change.

Communicate: Team Physicians Must Always be Available to Athletic Training Staff

If I were prioritizing these commandments, this one would rank near the top of the list. To build scholarship as well as your practice, develop a relationship with athletic trainers. Encourage them to ask the hard questions about injuries and to challenge you, the team physician, with questions. They can become close friends, but more importantly, they will definitely be members of your support team. Let the athletic trainers do their job on the field, meaning it's probably a mistake to run out to the middle of the field every time a player goes down. Wait for the athletic trainers to signal you.

In Order to Hit the Mark, One Must Aim a Little Higher

Everyone needs goals. Everyone has aspirations. But I have found that striving for a lofty goal is a better process than setting more limited, more achievable goals. Growing up, I enjoyed competing in any sport; however, I did not set my goals high enough. Like most of us team physicians, I was an athlete competing in any sport I could. I particularly enjoyed playing center forward on the field hockey team, but excelled in swimming. As a high school graduate of 1970, prior to Title IX, I was discouraged from swimming in college. I was lost without the structure swimming gave me. I made better grades and was more organized, not procrastinating when I was organized in the swimming. I continued to swim until almost all the way through medical school and retired in 1977 with a top 10 world ranking in breast stroke. I unsuccessfully tried out for the Olympics in 1972 and 1976 in swimming. I did not give up. On my third try, I made the Olympics as a US Olympic Committee team physician, in Barcelona in 1992.

Enjoy your Role as Team Physician

Be passionate about the opportunity to do what you love. Being a team physician is truly a privilege. Enjoy your time with team travel. Shopping is a good side benefit, and you always win at shopping despite what the football team may do. If you've got the tools to get through medical school and an orthopedic residency, then it's a good possibility that you didn't earn your position by complaining all the time. So if you foul something up, make the wrong call in a tense situation, and get your name in the paper under "Lawsuits Filed Today," the last thing you should do is complain to people about the problem you're having. Nobody ever feels sorry for you, and besides, as all politicians know, sooner or later it will all be forgotten. Life goes on.

Remember the five A's: Availability, Ability, Affability, Advocacy, Affiliation

Be available, able, and affable, affiliate with sports medicine associations, be an active member and be an advocate for your peers. I go to about 16 different meetings every year and I belong to several physician associations. Contributing to these organizations advances scholarship and research. It puts down roots with your colleagues in the field of sports medicine, and it networks all over the map. And when you need help yourself, either for a referral or maybe just a few words of advice and support from a friend, you will be glad you went through the hassle of air travel and hotel accommodations.

Human beings are fragile creatures with occasionally alarming and completely unpredictable psychological inclinations. Keeping your own act on an easily observable higher plane serves as a good role model to others, and late at night, allows the right sense of humility, self-awareness and, yes, balance to re-emerge.

Dare to Care

I have had the pleasure of working with three great long-term football coaches: Jerry Claiborne and Bill Curry at the University of Kentucky, and Roy Kidd at Eastern Kentucky University. These coaches truly cared about their players, families, and medical staff. They were like father figures to the players and taught these young men to be fine gentleman. These coaches instilled the goal of doing the right thing in the athletes. A football team is truly a family. The great coaches allowed me to direct the medical decisions and I let them coach—winning or losing! If I had been blessed with children, I would have been so proud for my sons to play for these great men. They never challenged the medical decisions.

My mother and father instilled in me their beliefs and commitments for me to respect and care and know right from wrong. Sports medicine is all about athletes; it is all about doing the right thing. Dare to care.

Don't Forget your Family and your Friends

I am not a parent, unless you count my beautiful Rhodesian Ridgeback (Belle) or my cats (Rascal and Thumper), or my husband, who thinks stubbing his toe is a near-death experience. But if you took the first nine of these so-called commandments and piled them up on one side of a balance pole, high above the center ring and with no net, this final one would easily bring the whole seesaw of life back to horizontal all by itself.

At the end of the day, we all have to go home. We all need a refuge, perhaps occasionally a shoulder to cry on.

My daddy died in 1992. I was called at the training room by my father's physician, who was at his bedside, and he told me to return quickly, that my father was going to die soon. Well, he died holding hands with his family on November 1, 1992—All Saints Day. Even in his last moments, he pressed my hand and wanted to know what he could do for me.

My mom is still here and I cherish every single minute I have left with her, and as I write these concluding words, I am sitting on my back porch on a cool, clear October afternoon in Kentucky. I can hear a high school band practicing off in the distance, and the leaves of the old sycamores in my backyard are turning to gold and swirling down one by one, and I do feel that my sense of balance is still here, never perfect, but still here, somewhere in the center of everything.

Clin Sports Med 26 (2007) 193–199

CLINICS IN SPORTS MEDICINE

EVIER
JNDERS

Negotiating Contractual Relationships

Charles Cole Nofsinger, MD, MS

Department of Orthopaedic Surgery, University of South Florida, 12901 Bruce B. Downs Boulevard, MDC 77, Tampa, FL 33612-4766, USA

Team physician is one of the most sought after positions in sports medicine. Surprisingly, only recently have the responsibilities of the team physician been defined by medical societies and athletic organizations that govern the parties involved. Many team physicians, in fact, do not have a contract with their team that defines the responsibilities of either party. The American Academy of Family Physicians (AAFP), American Academy of Orthopaedic Surgeons (AAOS), American College of Sports Medicine (ACSM), American Medical Society for Sports Medicine (AMSSM), American Orthopaedic Society for Sports Medicine (AOSSM), and the American Osteopathic Academy of Sports Medicine (AOASM) have developed a "Team Physician Consensus Statement" [1]. This statement delineates the responsibilities of the team physician. Likewise, the AOSSM has outlined the principles for selecting a team physician [2]. Unfortunately, Neither of these statements describes the contractual or financial relationship between the team and the physician. Yet the contract is a critical element in the long-term success of the relationship.

For many team physicians, the relationships are sealed with a verbal agreement and a handshake. In the majority of cases such verbal agreements have worked remarkably well. When they haven't worked well, athletes, physicians, and teams have suffered. Litigation of high-profile cases has raised awareness of the necessity for change. Although the structure of a contract needs to be individualized to the given situation, common elements and standards are being found as more teams formalize their relationships with the physicians that provide care and coverage.

A brief glimpse into the past puts the current situation into perspective. One of the first publicized cases of malpractice involving an athlete and his team physician occurred in 1975, when Dick Butkus sued the Chicago Bears of the National Football League (NFL) [3]. He alleged that the team physicians allowed him to play when the medical standard of care should have been to place him on bed rest. The suit was settled, but remarkably, the underlying conflict of interest that caused that suit has continued for at least 20 years.

E-mail address: cnofsing@health.usf.edu

0278-5919/07/$ – see front matter
doi:10.1016/j.csm.2007.01.010 © 2007 Elsevier Inc. All rights reserved.
sportsmed.theclinics.com

Recently changes made by the players associations, teams, and physician organizations have improved the care of professional athletes. The situation remains far from being straightforward.

Further examples of the types of concerns that exist with today's contractual relationships can be seen in the experiences of two very well-respected organizations. Before 2001, The Hospital for Special Surgery took care of the New York Mets Major League Baseball (MLB) club. That year the Mets asked the Hospital for Special Surgery for over one million dollars per year to continue as the team's physicians [4]. The hospital declined, based on ethical concerns. In turn, the New York University Hospital for Joint Disease bought the rights to be team physicians. The New York University hospital group provided physician coverage at no charge and received advertisements in Shea Stadium, game tickets, and personal visits from players at hospital events. In 2004, the Mets returned to the Hospital for Special Surgery as team physicians [5]. Now, The Hospital for Special Surgery is employed by the club to provide services and receives remuneration in return for their recognized skill set. The trend that had physicians and hospitals giving away services for free, and even in some cases paying millions of dollars to provide medical care, may be slowly reversing.

Professional athletes and their representatives have long recognized that medical coverage should be based solely on the quality of care. It is not unusual that an athlete's agent will dictate his or her medical care. In addition, the players' organizations help to define the access to care through the collective bargaining agreements. Without a doubt, there should be a well-defined responsibility for the physician to place the medical needs of the athlete above the needs of the team. Yet this runs counter to the inherent team-oriented mind set of athletes who often desire a quick, short-term solution that may not be in their best interests. The team physician must maintain an impartial perspective on the health of the athlete despite concerns over the implication of his contractual arrangements.

This impartiality is challenged by the financial arrangement many physicians have with their professional teams. The NFL has a position statement that requires physicians not pay their teams [6]. The NFL collective bargaining agreement [7] requires the team to pay for medical care; however, it does not require that team physicians be employees of the team. It can be beneficial to the physician to be employed, because it limits the liability of the team physician under worker's compensation. If a team physician is not an employee, he or his organization may have liability for financial loss of wages. For a professional athlete, that could reach into the tens of millions of dollars, far beyond the scope of most malpractice coverages.

This has led to a crisis in malpractice coverage for team physicians, just as there is for physicians in private practice. The crisis varies by the state in which you practice. For example, in Wisconsin there is an unlimited worker's compensation pool that protects professional team physicians, whereas in Pennsylvania, there is no compensation pool, and increasingly only university-based physicians are able to cover teams without going bare (operating without malpractice insurance).

Dr. Andrew Bishop, one time Atlanta Falcons team physician, has been quoted as saying that there are three options: "(1) have physicians become employees of their respective leagues, (2) have physicians become employees of the players association, or (3) have a panel of qualified physicians who understand the demands of team physicians serve as a litigation qualifying board for any player thinking about suing" [8]. In fact, physician organizations have approached the NFL, National Basketball Association (NBA), MLB, and National Hockey League (NHL) about this issue. To the author's knowledge, none of the leagues have negotiated such a deal.

Many players' organizations have guaranteed impartial medical care for their players by placing appropriate clauses in their collective bargaining agreements [8]. These agreements outline the team's responsibilities to the player, and by so doing also stipulate the role of the physician. Consider the following from the MLB collective bargaining agreement:

> C. Disabled List
> Application by a Club to the Commissioner to place a Player on the Disabled List shall be accompanied by a Standard Form of Diagnosis. This Standard Form of Diagnosis shall be completed by the Club physician and shall include, as a separate item, an estimated time period for recovery. A copy of the completed Standard Form will be given to the Player and the Association. The Club physician will also complete and submit the Standard Form of Diagnosis for recertification of a Player on the Disabled List at the date when he first becomes eligible for reinstatement to active status and then every fifteen days following the date upon which the Player first became eligible for reinstatement (except for Players placed upon the Emergency Disabled List).
> Section XIX
> (1) There shall be no assignment of a Player by a Major League Club to a Minor League club while such Player is on a Major League Disabled List; provided, however, that with the Player's written consent, a copy of which shall be forwarded to the Association, and with the approval of the Commissioner, a Player on the Disabled List may be assigned to a Minor League club for up to a maximum of twenty days (thirty days for pitchers) for each injury, or reoccurrence of an injury, for the purpose of rehabilitation, subject to the limits contained in Article XIII(H). Separate consent shall be required for a rehabilitation assignment for a new injury or a reoccurrence of an injury. No consent shall be effective for longer than twenty days (thirty days for pitchers).

Failure of the physician to understand these rules could have consequences not only for the physician but for the team and the player. Physicians may be asked to inappropriately keep a player on the disabled list. With large pay loss possible, physicians may be sued if their behavior is determined to be extreme, and this makes understanding the contractual requirements key to the awareness of the business aspect of providing health care. Consider this extract from the NFL collective bargaining agreement:

> Section 1. Club Physician: Each Club will have a board-certified orthopedic surgeon as one of its Club physicians. The cost of medical services rendered by Club physicians will be the responsibility of the respective Clubs. If a Club physician advises a coach or other Club representative of a player's physical condition which adversely affects the player's performance or health, the physician will also advise the player. If such condition could be significantly aggravated by continued performance, the physician will advise the player of such fact in writing before the player is again allowed to perform on-field activity.

Note the ambiguity of the condition that the patient be advised in writing. What does "significantly aggravated" mean? Again, the team physician must be conversant with the requirements of the governing body. There are many professional team physicians for the NFL and the MLB that do not have contracts. Despite having no contracts, their behavior is still governed by the collective bargaining agreements, in essence forming a contractual responsibility. Understanding your responsibilities requires diligence and most likely, legal counsel.

Obviously, contractual relationships with teams are of the utmost importance to the physician, the athlete, the team and the governing body. What follows is a discussion of the specific elements of the contract:

- Parties discussed in the contract
- Responsibilities of the physician organization
- Responsibilities of the team
- Term of the contract

PARTIES DISCUSSED

The principal parties are the team, the athlete, and the physician. There are many more people involved in the actual care of athletes, and these parties are also usually mentioned. Coaches, for instance, may be included for the same level of care as the athletes. Athletic trainers and physical therapists may have a defined level of care provided by the team. The level of insurance coverage and the insurance companies may also be stipulated. Most professional athletes are covered by state worker's compensation laws. Although there is precedent for collegiate athletes receiving coverage under worker's compensation, collegiate athletes are not considered eligible by default [9]. A collegiate contract may require that the university carry appropriate health insurance for its student athletes to pay for appropriate health care.

As evidenced above in the collective bargaining agreement, the player's association, the team, and the governing bodies together regulate medical care. Because of the multiple requirements, it may be difficult to comply. Therefore, most contracts will contain a clause stating that the contract attempts to comply with the rules of the governing body. If, however, the contract is found to be in violation of the other rules, the contract is amended to comply.

To control fees, a physician group may agree to use certain medical treatment, imaging, testing, and physical therapy facilities. This is not in conflict with the AOSSM position statement on team medical coverage, because it specifically allows for flexibility in financial matters; however, it does encourage full disclosure. In addition, all collective bargaining agreements have a means for an athlete to get a second opinion that is paid for by the team.

PHYSICIAN RESPONSIBILITIES

It is the physicians', responsibility to be appropriately certified and licensed to care for the athletes. In addition, physicians must carry malpractice insurance at a level appropriate to the athlete. This can be very expensive for coverage of professional athletes. In some states this may mean that only university groups are able to afford coverage.

Physician responsibilities may include more than just the care of the injured athlete. Contracts will stipulate the amount of coverage and also whether primary care, orthopedic, or other coverage is included. For professional and college sports, on-field coverage of every game is typically provided with revenue-generating and spectator sports such as football and basketball. Risk of injury and gender equality should also be considered. Some contracts may allow the team physician to designate another physician to act as team physician for a specific game. Contracts also specify pre-participation clearance duties, and perhaps other oversight of clinical policies and procedures, such as medication dispensation, concussion management, and environmental emergencies, to include heat-related illnesses. Contracts do not typically cover consultation and treatment staff beyond the coaching staff. Many physicians will cover the staff as a courtesy, but it is wise to see the patients in your regular office setting to avoid "curbside" consult care. Curbside consultations are much more prevalent in athletics populations, including coaches, staff members, and extended families.

Pre-participation clearance is especially pertinent to professional sports, where large salaries are paid based on the fitness and performance abilities of the athlete. It is essential that a team physician understand his responsibility to examine and document every detail of a professional athlete injury encounter. Failure to discover an injury can have significant legal ramifications, not to mention the fiscal loss and individual/team performance concerns. There are standard forms for documentation that have been agreed upon by all parties [10].

Contracts may stipulate that physicians give team members priority service. The fee for service may also be stipulated by the contract. This may be a flat fee, but the contract will usually stipulate that fees be only the customary amount and no more. Regardless, careful attention to detail and learning from consultation and the experience of others is invaluable.

TEAM RESPONSIBILITIES

The contract should stipulate that the team will designate the physician organization the official team physicians in all media. The contract may or may not stipulate that the athlete is required to use that organization for their primary medical coverage. Most organizations reserve the right for their players to see any physician or get a second opinion above and beyond the collective bargaining agreements.

The team should be responsible for providing appropriate insurance. At the college level, the students' primary insurance is provided by their families and secondary insurance is provided by the university; however, many do not have primary insurance, and there is no guarantee of the acceptance of such insurance with many players at an institution outside the state of the provided coverage. Most professional teams provide coverage through worker's compensation. At the high school level, the school may or may not provide insurance if the family has none. It is the choice of each physician as to how he will address the patient with no insurance.

The team should provide appropriate clothing in order for the physician to represent the team. Above and beyond that, the team may provide clothing and merchandise to help the physician advertise the association. These are all negotiable points that will indirectly assist the physician with marketing efforts within his or her own practice setting.

The team should provide appropriate training room facilities and the appropriate number of certified athletic trainers to treat the athletes on a day-to-day basis. Few physicians could cover teams without certified athletic trainers. The certified athletic trainer is a key element to the relationship among the athlete, coach, and physician. It is important to understand the implications of level of athletic trainer coverage. A high school with no athletic trainer will require much more of the physician's time. At the professional and college level, it is critical that there be adequate athletic trainers available to care for all off- and on-field needs of the athlete.

The team should provide appropriate equipment and supplies, including braces, padding, medical supplies, instruments, injectables, and medications for the team physician to appropriately care for the team's athletes. Communication in advance, "dry-runs," and thorough planning will assist tremendously in being prepared for the supply needs of sideline and training room care.

Finally, the team should reimburse all travel costs or provide travel to and from practices and games.

TERMS OF CONTRACT

Marketing rules are typically specified that determine how each party may use the logo of the other. Typically each side must obtain consent before public use of the other party's trademarked or patented logo.

The duration of an agreement may vary from 1 year to many. The contract may be terminated for breach, usually after written notice only.

Both parties typically agree to be bound by the intent of the governing body in case the contract unknowingly conflicts with the regulations of the governing body.

SUMMARY

Establishing a contractual relationship with a team may not be a negotiation. Most teams are highly sought after. Evaluate the realistic risks and benefits of covering a team, however. Herb Cohen, a negotiator for governments and companies, has said that you should care about negotiating a deal, but not that much. Understand what the team is looking for. Prior physicians may have been dismissed because of a specific action, they may have left on their own, or they may have been asked to pay for the privilege of being a team physician. Finally, tell the team what you have to offer and what you need to make the relationship work, and be prepared to walk away from the deal if the risks are too high.

Team coverage can be the most rewarding and the most challenging aspect of a physician's career. Understanding the implications of working without a contract and the elements of an appropriate contract are paramount to a successful relationship.

References

[1] Team physician consensus statement. 2001.

[2] Principles for selecting team medical coverage. AOSSM; 2005.

[3] George T. Care by team doctors raises conflict issue. New York Times. July 28, 2002.

[4] Beaton R. Medical staff moves prompt questions. USA Today. October 21, 2001.

[5] Anderson S. Is there a doctor in the clubhouse? Pittsburgh Post-Gazette. October 10, 2004.

[6] Tagliabue P. Memo on hospital and physician sponsorships. NFL news release. September 7, 2004.

[7] National football league collective bargaining agreement. Available at: http://www.nflpa. org/CBA/CBA.aspx. Accessed February 2007.

[8] Kober S. Team physicians questioning their future. Orthopaedics Today. September, 2002.

[9] J Law and Education, Oct 2001.

[10] Major League Baseball. Collective bargaining agreement. Available at: http://mlbplayers. mlb.com/pa/pdf/cba_english.pdf. Accessed February 2007.

Clin Sports Med 26 (2007) 201–226

CLINICS IN SPORTS MEDICINE

SEVIER
JNDERS

Understanding Organization Structures of the College, University, High School, Clinical, and Professional Settings

Mike Goforth, MS, ATC[a], Jon Almquist, MS, ATC[b],
Martin Matney, MBA, MS, ATC, PTA[c],
Thomas E. Abdenour, MA, ATC[d], James Kyle, MD[e],
Joe Leaman, MS, ATC[f], Scott Montgomery, MD[g],*

[a]Virginia Tech University, Eddie Ferrell Athletic Training Facility, 160 Jamerson Athletic Center, Blacksburg, VA 24061, USA
[b]Fairfax County Public Schools, Athletic Training Program, 8115 Gatehouse Road, Suite 5100, Falls Church, VA 22042, USA
[c]Whitesel ProTherapy, Inc., 13120 NE 70th Place, Suite 3, Kirkland, WA 98033, USA
[d]Golden State Warriors, 1011 Broadway, Oakland, CA 94607, USA
[e]Family, Athletic and Recreational Medicine, 1101 A1A, Ponte Vedra, FL 32082, USA
[f]HEALTHSOUTH Sports Medicine and Rehabilitation Center, 2200 Grand Central Ave. #A, Vienna, WV 36101, USA
[g]Ochsner Sports Medicine, 1514 Jefferson Highway, New Orleans, LA 70121, USA

Athletes participate at many different levels of competition—from amateur to professional, from backyard sandlot to Yankee Stadium. There are as many different organized structures involved in providing medical care to athletes as there are types of athletes themselves. Although the organizational structures involved in providing medical care for a little league team in a small town are different from those involved in providing care for a professional baseball team, the mission is the same—caring for athletes. This is the central theme of this article. Though there are different organizational structures, there are more common threads than differences in the mission of those who provide medical care for athletes at any level.

One of the key components to providing care to athletes is to understand the inherent expectations of the population for which you are caring. Understanding the resources that you have available to care for your athletes is equally important. Providing effective care of athletes or teams at any level starts with two common pillars: good personnel and an organized, thought-out plan of care.

Good personnel might seem too obvious to mention, but they are the backbone of sports medicine as a field and are critical when caring for athletes.

*Corresponding author. E-mail address: scmontgo@hotmail.com (S. Montgomery).

0278-5919/07/$ – see front matter
doi:10.1016/j.csm.2007.01.005
© 2007 Elsevier Inc. All rights reserved.
sportsmed.theclinics.com

Central to this idea is relationship building. When consideration is given to either hiring a new member of a sports medicine team or allowing a person or group to provide care for an athlete or team, some important factors should be weighed. First, is the person qualified and capable of providing adequate care for the athletes involved? Second, and no less important, is to determine the person's ability to relate to the athlete, coaches, managers, athletic trainers, and other physicians, as well as team personnel. The interpersonal skills considered important in being a good professional and a good person are even more important for a physician or athletic trainer wishing to care for athletes at any level. Third is the person's honest appraisal of his or her own abilities. Team physicians are now often not the only member of an athletes' total care package, and proper standard of care now quite frequently involves coordinating visits to other health care professionals. The days of stubborn paternalism have gone the way of football players playing both offense and defense, as more and more subspecialization enters the medical field. Though this adds more complexity to an organization taking care of an athletic team, it can provide a higher level of care for its athletes. In short, a good team physician has to be technically and mentally capable, personally dedicated and engaging, and professionally humble enough to ensure proper care for the athletes under his or her care.

An organized, thought-through plan of care is the second important piece of effectively caring for athletes at any level. A common perception of team physicians is that they are present on the sidelines at various sporting events. Although this is an integral part of caring for many athletes in contact sports such as lacrosse, ice hockey, and football, it is only part of a total plan of care for athletes and teams. To effectively care for any large group of people, attention must be paid early in the process for all members of the organization to communicate with each other the following three ideas: (1) the level of expectations, (2) the proper roles for the various personnel involved, and (3) contingency planning. It has been the authors' experience that the earlier all parties come to an understanding about the details of all three of these ideas, the more effective the care becomes.

Not all athletic team structures are the same. A youth soccer league is quite different from a National Collegiate Athletic Association (NCAA) Division I-AA football program, and the level of expectations for medical coverage is understandably not the same. An approach to providing care for these athletes can follow a similar template though, and this begins with setting the expectation level. The volunteer youth soccer league director might be upset if he assumes that an athletic trainer or physician will be attending every Saturday all-day soccer marathon if the expectation level is not set early on that medical care will be available but not present at every event. The I-AA football coach could become equally confrontational if athletic trainer coverage but not physician coverage were provided at spring practices, if this was not his expectation. Both scenarios could be avoided by communication and early establishment of the levels of expectation of all parties involved.

It is equally important to establish the proper role of each member of the medical team well in advance of team competition. Smaller communities with one orthopedic surgeon and one athletic trainer covering all of the athletes for the local high school will likely have a broad mandate to provide or coordinate all of the care for the athletes they see and treat. A large university setting or a professional team in a large metropolitan area provides a different environment for team physicians and athletic trainers to treat their athletes. In this setting, multiple providers and health care systems are available, and are in close proximity to the teams and their athletes; the proper roles and referral patterns can be confusing if not clearly delineated well ahead of time. Again, the answer to this problem is establishing clear roles for the decision-making in the organization, whether that involves one person or a team of people.

Contingency planning is critically important to any corporate organization, and medical care for an athlete should not be treated any differently. Before the season starts, the organization managers and the medical team should go through a series of "what if" scenarios: What if lightning is seen in the area of our football game?; What if the team physician cannot attend a game because of a family emergency?; What if a home lacrosse game and a visiting football game are conducted simultaneously for the same university staff?; and so forth. Most potential conflicts can be easily resolved ahead of time if the proper legwork is done before the season.

Another key component for any organization providing medical care for athletes is to adapt to changes in a positive way. As anyone who keeps up with the medical literature knows, there is an explosion of new scientific information that can be applied directly to the medical care of our athletes. Whether it involves bracing knees for medial collateral ligament injury prevention, proper pitch counts for youth baseball, screening for sickle trait before August football, or treatment options for athletic pubalgia from our general surgery colleagues, keeping up to date and properly applying the current medical information can help optimize the care and thus performance of our athletes.

An organization can facilitate change in ways that are involved with organizational structure, but that can still directly improve athletic care. This might involve improving a group of university athletes' access to a medical provider, whether primary care, orthopedic surgeon, or other specialist. This can often involve a scheduled time in an athletic training room (whether daily or weekly) when athletes and athletic trainers will have direct access to primary care and specialist team physicians. This might also involve a local hospital providing personnel for a Saturday morning walk-in clinic to better serve the needs of local high school football players.

Being a team physician provides many challenges that differ depending on the level of athlete and team being covered. As anyone who has cared for young athletes knows, one of the biggest challenges in amateur sports medicine care is effective communication with and reliable follow-through from the parents and coaches of these future All-Americans. When caring for these young athletes with whom you have limited contact, such as only in office visits or in pre-partic-ipation physicals, effective preventative strategies are difficult but vital to pro-mote. Maintaining a tactful balance between the desires of the involved parent, the overbearing coach, and the high-pain-tolerance, traveling-team youth athlete is often a challenge whose difficulty is underappreciated. As always, the most im-portant role of a team physician in this setting is to be an advocate for the young athlete and put his or her health as the top priority.

The team physician in a university setting experiences a different set of chal-lenges. In addition to the desires of parents and team coaches of youth sports, there is now an even higher level of expectations from teams and programs for athletes to play through injuries when on-field victories create job security for coaches. Athletes at this level or higher have focused their participation in one sport, and some have begun to think of their bodies and skills as a potential income generator in the near future. Medical decision-making in this setting must involve an open communication line between athletes, coaches, athletic trainers, physicians, and parents, so that all parties are on the same page as to the reasons behind any treatment plan developed by the medical staff. Espe-cially at this level of competition or higher, return-to- play issues must be con-templated and addressed as early as possible.

The team physician for a professional team juggles the same set of challenges as one in a university setting, but with several added factors. The athlete's body has now become his or her source of income, and medical decision-making will likely have an impact on the athlete's ability to compete at the desired level. In addition to coaches and family, agents, team owners, and contracts are now fac-tors in the athlete's response to his or her injury, and pressure exists for them to play a role in treatment recommendation.

A physician's primary role is to be an advocate for his or her patient. The cen-tral mission of a team physician, then, is to care for athletes at each of these levels of competition in exactly the same way—to be the athlete's advocate above all else. Making the best medical decision for an injured athlete often involves facing strong pressures from different outside parties whose goals might not include what is judged to be in the athlete's best interest. It is precisely in these situations that the experience and judgment of a good team physician is most important.

ORGANIZATIONAL STRUCTURE OF THE TEAM PHYSICIAN IN A HIGH SCHOOL SETTING

The physician serving as a team physician in a high school is faced with a variety of responsibilities, depending on the circumstances that exist in that unique setting. There are two basic organizational structures that present in the high school: a situation in which the school employs the services of a certi-fied athletic trainer who is available on site on a daily basis and is responsible for the athletic health care of all student athletes, and another in which there is no medically educated health care provider available to the student athletes. Before delving into the specifics of each situation, there are some components of the team physician relationship that are consistent between both structures.

There are many benefits awarded to the physician who commits to being a high school team physician. Providing a community service and being available as a role model for many students each year is of great value. It is a marketing opportunity that will help attract sports medicine-related cases, not only with high school athletes, but also for weekend warriors and the general physically active community, because the physician is visible on the field and court during games, with spectators packing the stands. The marketing opportunity extends to increased patient load overall, because family members of high school athletes may also be in search of medical services.

The services a team physician should expect to provide to a high school include providing pre-participation physical examinations pursuant to the school division or state athletic conference requirements, providing return-to-participation criteria following an injury, and providing medical care without charge for student athletes with financial hardships when appropriate.

When the physician is the only medically trained person available at a high school, responsibilities may include everything from basic first aid during contests to sports medicine-related educational programs such as hydration protocols, sports-related nutrition programs, injury prevention strategies, return-to-play decisions, concussion evaluation, skin disorder diagnosis, and so forth. It is important to understand that the team physician must take a comprehensive approach to the athletic health care of all student athletes within a school.

The services a team physician should expect to provide to a high school will be significantly different with the availability of an on-site athletic health care provider such as a certified athletic trainer. An on-site health care provider available at the school on a daily basis changes the role of the team physician considerably. The certified athletic trainer will be responsible for serving as the athletic health coordinator under the direction of a team physician, as described in the American Medical Association (AMA) resolution H-470.995, "Athletic (Sports) Medicine," published in 1998. The certified athletic trainer should be responsible for providing first aid not only during games, but also for practices throughout the season. The certified athletic trainer should also be able to care for and develop treatment plans for the majority of issues that he or she is presented with. In the event of a more significant injury, such as a suspected fracture, the athlete should be referred to a physician. In most high school situations, the responsibility for a student's medical care lies with the parents, so the parents will choose which physician they take their child to. In suburban areas, the choice of physician can be vast, and the team physician will need to be sensitive to the professional political climate. The team physician can act as a second opinion in some cases when the family's choice of treating physician may not be well-versed in sports medicine or sports-related injuries.

Working the Sidelines with a Certified Athletic Trainer

What is the team physician's role on the sideline when working with a certified athletic trainer? One thing to consider is that the certified athletic trainer most likely knows the athletes, their personalities, demeanors, and pain tolerances much better than the team physician, who may only see the athletes on a very brief basis. The certified athletic trainer is well-educated in the provision of first aid, protection of an injury with creative protective devices, and sport-specific assessment of functional status.

Confirming the conformational diagnosis, facilitating follow-up laboratory test or tests such as radiographs, MRIs, and the like can be a primary function and benefit of having a physician on the sidelines. This also provides a tremendous opportunity for discussion of all the cases that were presented during the week.

The majority of injuries that occur when a physician is present (at a game) fall into the minor bumps, sprains, and strains category. The challenge in dealing with these types of injuries on the sidelines is determination of the return to play in that game. Past experiences have demonstrated that many physicians don't have much experience with evaluating musculoskeletal injuries acutely (within minutes) in a way that coincides with the rules and speed of the sport.

Team Physician Role Throughout the Year

Providing an opportunity to evaluate athletes at the school during the week can be a tremendous advantage to a school, with or without a certified athletic trainer on site at the school on a regular basis. Discuss the benefits of providing an expedited appointment mechanism and the need to have the office staff in tune to who from the school will be calling to see if an athlete can be seen within the next hour or day.

ORGANIZATIONAL STRUCTURES OF THE COLLEGE AND UNIVERSITY SETTINGS

The landscape of college athletics has changed dramatically over the course of the last 15 years. For better or worse, the structure of intercollegiate athletics has changed from mere athletic competition to a year-round enterprise potentially generating millions of dollars for colleges and universities across the country. With this increased intensity comes increased pressure and expectations by all of the involved staff members responsible for recruiting, training, and caring for our number one resource, the athlete.

Fifteen years ago the typical medical staff associated with the college or university setting was relatively small, with very little diversity in training and a lack of involvement in many of the sports outside of the traditional football and men's and women's basketball. Typically schools had a head athletic trainer, at least two or three assistant athletic trainers, and a primary care physician or an orthopedic surgeon. Because of the small staff sizes, many staffs were limited in what they could provide and cover. Over time, increased athletic expectations for coverage and services far exceeded increases in staff sizes. Increased awareness of the health care needs of the athletes led athletic administrators across the country to assign a higher priority to increasing not only the size, but also the scope of sports medicine services.

Many of today's larger institutions have a multitude of health care providers to meet the needs of their athletes. The challenge facing today's athletic department is how to manage the many resources at its disposal to provide sound medical care and establish an environment that balances the need for growth with the needs of the competitive athlete.

In considering the delivery of medical care to NCAA Division I athletes, author Goforth conducted a survey on the authors' behalf to identify the following variables as areas that need to be considered when assessing the organizational structure of the college or university health care delivery system:

1. Academic discipline of staff members
2. Medical and administrative oversight of staff members
3. Employment agreement structures of staff members
4. Athlete access to sports medicine services

During the spring of 2006, author Goforth surveyed 89 Division I sports medicine departments and asked full-time staff members the following questions to help the authors understand the above-mentioned variables:

1. How many primary care physicians do you use in your department?
2. How many orthopedic physicians do you use in your department?
3. How many fellows or residents do you use in your department?
4. Do you identify a head team physician, and if so, is he or she a primary care physician or an orthopedic physician?
5. Do you use any dictated referral patterns such as requiring that the athlete see the primary care physician before the orthopedic physician?
6. Do any of your physicians work through student health?
7. Do any of your physicians work through your medical school?

The results of the survey are summarized by athletic conference in Table 1.

Discipline and Certification of Staff Members

Across the nation, there is a great emphasis on the provision of medical care to athletes. There are numerous organizational structures. There were numerous anecdotal references during the survey to the academic conflicts between primary care and orthopedic specialties regarding who was best qualified to care for the athlete. To further the controversy, there now exists additional training in "sports medicine" fellowships within both primary care and orthopedics. In a search of the literature, countless editorials have been written with opinions on who is best suited to provide care to collegiate athletes. Only one published article was found to provide data on team physician preferences at NCAA Division I universities. In 1997, Dr. Stockard [1] published the results of a survey investigating the specialty and qualification of current team physicians at NCAA Division I universities, along with the preferences of athletic directors as to what specialty of physician they would most like to have working with their respective departments. The results of the study revealed several key points that warrant additional research and serve as a good source of information for administrators to use for future hiring purposes. In that survey, the majority of team physicians were

Table 1
Results of phone survey of Division I sports medicine programs. A summary of results for each conference is listed below.

Conference[a]	PCP #[b]	Ortho #[b]	Fellow #[b]	Head[c]	Referral pattern[d]	SH[e]	Med[e]
Mt. West N = 2	3	5	0	2 O	0	0	0
A-10/Colonial N = 7	10.5	15	4	6 P	0	3	1
Big 12 N = 12	36	40	4	6 P, 5 O	0	8	2
Big South N = 4	5	8	0	2 P, 2 O	0	2	0
OVC N = 2	4	5	0	0 P, 1 O	0	0	0
Southern N = 11	16	23	4	1 P, 6 O	0	6	0
Big East N = 8	15	21	13	4 P, 4 O	0	3	2
C-USA N = 9	22	30	18	5 P, 3 O	0	5	3
MAC N = 6	8	12	7	4 O	0	1	1
IND. N = 1	3	5	2	Co	0	1	0
ACC N = 12	31	32	9	4 P, 5 O	0	4	4
Pac-10 N = 4	11	15	9	2 P, 2 O	0	3	1
Big 10 N = 11	32	32	14	3 P, 4 O	2	4	2
Total N = 89	196.5	243	84	33 P, 39 O	2	40	16

Abbreviations: A-10/Colonial, Atlantic Ten/Colonial; ACC, Atlantic Coast Conference; C-USA, Conference USA; IND, Independents; MAC, Mid Atlantic Conference; Med, medical school; Mt. West, Mountain West; N, number; O, orthopedists; OVC, Ohio Valley Conference; P, primary care specialist; Pac-10, Pacific Ten; SH, student health.

[a]Number of teams contacted in each conference is indicated.

[b]The table shows the number of primary care specialists (PCP), orthopedists (Ortho) and fellows for the programs contacted.

[c]Head team physician is listed by specialty.

[d]Mandated referral patterns from athletic trainers to specific physician are as listed.

[e]Affiliations with student Health or Medical Schools for the provision of medical care are summarized.

primary care and orthopedic surgeons, with a relatively small number of team physicians coming from the areas of pediatrics, internal medicine, neurology, general surgery, and physical medicine and rehabilitation.

Author Goforth's survey looked at the differences in the specialties of physicians used. Survey respondents reported the number of primary care physicians and the number of orthopedic physicians used in their respective departments. The results revealed that schools had an average 2.2 primary care physicians and 2.7 orthopedic physicians. Only one school reported using an internal medicine physician, and one reported using a pediatrician as the team physician; no schools reported using a neurologist as one of their team physicians. The survey also revealed that 39% of the schools were using fellows or residents to supplement the services offered by the team physician. The discipline of the fellow was largely dependent on the specialty of the identified head team physician.

Medical and Administrative Oversight of Staff Members

Each person involved in the provision of sports medicine services within the organization should have a comprehensive personnel file. This file should begin with an objective job description outlining the scope of services, as well as a chain of command identifying where the person fits within the organizational structure on clinical and administrative levels. In addition, the employee or volunteer should also have some form of documentation (contract or letter of agreement) of the appointment as a provider of services, the length of the appointment, and by whom the appointment was made. The file should also contain copies of all licenses and certifications necessary to practice in the respective setting. In the survey, author Goforth found that 16 of 89 schools had contractual agreements with a medical school or student health service for the provision of medical care.

Contractual issues are important because they not only establish expectations and responsibilities, but they can also help to prevent or minimize conflict. Goforth's survey incidentally identified frequent conflicts arising between physicians and athletic personnel with regard to who directs the care of the athlete. One school reported that problems between physicians led to the dismissal of one team physician. A second school reported that problems between physicians led to the resignation of the head athletic trainer. These issues have drawn the attention of athletic conferences and are being addressed on a conference level in hopes of preventing further incidents.

Head Team Physicians

There is a debate across the country surrounding who should be the head team physician. This debate occurs on a daily bases in training programs, editorials, and Web-based list serves, and is based on biases such as discipline and training type. The survey revealed that 37% of the schools reported naming the primary care physician as the head team physician, 43% named the orthopedic physician as the head team physician, and 20% of the schools do not identify any physician as their head team physician. The survey revealed a general sense in training rooms across the country that previously the "team physician" had a very loosely defined relationship built on mutual respect and a strong desire to serve the institution. Now, it appears to be a more highly competitive and sought-after title. This underscores the importance of proactively developing institutional structure and organization for the provision of medical services. This structure and organization should be reviewed annually.

Employment Agreement Structures of Staff Members

As stated earlier, all support personnel should have some type of formal arrangement with their respective institution. This documentation is usually in the form of a contract or letter of agreement signed off on by the athletic director of the institution. There are currently four models used on the collegiate level: (1) full-time private practice physician working with a team, (2) full- or part-time physician working between the athletic department and student health services, (3) full- or part-time physician working between the athletic department and a medical school, and (4) physicians employed on a full-time basis within the athletic department. The survey revealed that 44% of the schools used physicians with dual appointments between student health services and the athletic department, and 16% of the school used physicians with dual appointments between a medical school and the athletic department. Whether full-time, part-time, or dually appointed, it is very important that duties and expectations be clearly outlined to prevent misunderstandings by the multiple departments over the physician's time and expertise.

Athlete Access to Sports Medicine Services

Access to sports medicine services will be determined by facility size, institutional philosophy, facility availability, physician availability, and athlete availability. Access to physician services can either be made through self referral from the athlete or by referral from one of the school's certified athletic trainers. Most institutions use the certified athletic trainer referral system to filter certain cases as well as to maintain open lines of communication among the athlete, coaches, certified athletic trainers, and physicians.

Once the referral pattern has been established, the next consideration is how the physician visit is structured. Currently two models exist: the clinic model and the appointment model. The clinic model is used with a set location and time for the physician to see whoever has been referred. The physician is at the mercy of how many patients have been referred, and sees patients on a first-come, first-see basis. Typically the clinics are in the morning before classes or in the evenings after practice. The appointment model uses set days, times, and appointment time slots for each patient encounter (eg, appointment slots every 10 minutes). Attention should be paid to insure that the proper amount of time is allocated for certain procedures that routinely take longer, such as physicals and small procedures. In those situations, care should be taken to book multiple time slots.

Two areas of note that warrant additional programming and planning are in the areas of specialty referrals and communication. Author Goforth's phone survey revealed an increased concern over referral patterns. The conflict arises over who is best suited to care for a certain type of injury. Much like the conflict over naming a head team physician, conflict is developing between sports medicine primary care physicians and orthopedic physicians, and is debated on many different levels across various media. Strict policies and protocols that outline the direction of referrals and how these referrals will be communicated between physicians must be drafted and agreed upon by all parties before each school year . The plan of care for an athlete should not be compromised because of ego-related issues; this only delays proper care and sends mixed signals to the injured athlete. The survey indicated that 2 out of 89 schools had dictated referral patterns. These 2 schools requested that all injuries see the primary care physician before any further referral, such as to an orthopedic physician. Of note, one of the school's policies were based on the fact that the orthopedic physician was located in a different city that required travel time and set clinic hours. The overwhelming majority of the respondents stated that the referral was a judgment call by the certified athletic trainer, and usually followed the rationale of illnesses referred to the primary care physician and injuries to bone and joints referred to the orthopedic physician. Many of the referrals were also based on physician availability and who was available at the onset of the condition. Many of the respondents stated that they considered the availability, personality style, and management style of the physician over any one type of training or discipline. Interestingly, one school surveyed has a formal annual meeting in which all parties set down before each school year and discuss referral patterns among physicians to insure consistency and communication.

Future Directions

For all of the questions that the survey tried to answer, it is increasingly evident that additional research needs to be conducted in this area. Each of the five variables needs to be dissected and a more comprehensive survey developed to investigate each area in greater detail. One variable that was not looked at in the survey is the role of board certification and fellowship training. Advanced training and certification may be a more important variable than the individual's medical discipline. In addition, the survey did not explore osteopathic or allopathic specialization of team physicians. A third weakness of the survey is that it did not investigate the use of additional providers, including chiropractors and sport psychologists. Chiropractic and sport psychologists services are being employed on a much more frequent basis across the country in the college and university settings. The organizational structure of these services needs further investigation. The authors suspect that detailed policies and procedures for these services are organized in much the same way as other physician services.

No matter how big the area of sports medicine gets, it is important that we always consider our respective roles within the institution we work at and within the lives of our athletes. Team physicians play a tremendous role in Division I athletics and serve to protect our greatest asset, the athlete. Their role and value can never be underestimated or overappreciated, and we owe them a great deal of respect and gratitude.

CLINICAL SETTING

As in a physician's office, a clinical rehabilitation setting focuses on the injured individual. In the clinical setting the injured athlete in effect becomes a client or patient. This discussion refers to this person as the "patient/athlete."

The clinical setting presents a variety of interrelated yet unique relationships among numerous stakeholders. These affiliations ultimately revolve around the patient/athlete, and include the team physician; the health care provider, such as the athletic trainer or physical therapist; and clinical staff, including front office personnel, billing staff, and ancillary employees. An unseen entity in the relationship between the team physician and the patient/athlete is the clinic owner, be it an individual directly involved in patient care, an ownership entity such as investors or multiclinic ownership groups, or a corporate institution. At times, the team physician may have an economic interest in the clinical facility, but this is less common than it was many years ago.

A clinical facility is generally a for-profit entity. As such, its purpose is to provide care to the patient/athlete in a cost-effective manner, and to maximize the effectiveness of each visit to deliver proper care and contribute to the return of the patient/athlete to his or her sport. Each person employed in this facility at different times provides assistance to the patient/athlete, but most often this care should be overseen by a primary care-giver. This person should be that team's athletic trainer, or at the very least, the health care provider who cares for the team or school. In some cases, most often because of insurance limitations or locale, the patient/athlete will receive care at a clinical facility that has no direct ties to his or her school or group. In this case, it is best that the team athletic trainer or team physician have contact with this particular facility and establish communication with the person providing the care to the patient/athlete in order to coordinate care and facilitate return to activity.

Clinical health care to athletes often is a result of an outreach program, with staff sent from the clinic to the school or team. This staff should be qualified, such as an appropriately credentialed athletic trainer, and the team physician should be aware of the background of the person caring for these athletes. If there is any question as to the medical preparedness of this individual, the team physician should address this with clinic management, because it is this person that the team physician relies on for the immediate care and proper referral of these athletes.

The clinical outreach program is often used as a referral tool for the clinic, with injured athletes often receiving their rehabilitative care at the clinic. The team physician fits into this loop as the physician the athlete is most often referred to for initial physician care. This referral to physician is usually conducted by the attending clinic staff, such as the clinic athletic trainer assigned to that team. The team athletic trainer may see the injured athlete on the field, in the training room, or even in the clinic. Wherever the athlete is seen, it is up to the person seeing him or her to conduct a proper evaluation, initiate treatment, and refer the patient to the team physician.

The clinical setting is unlike the collegiate, university, or professional training room. Here, a patient/athlete will often receive rehabilitation next to non-athletes and the so-called "general public." Unlike other training rooms, team physician contact is limited unless the physician regularly visits the clinic or the patient/athlete sees the physician on a scheduled office call. Occasionally, the team physician may see the athlete at the school training room or on the field, and may conduct an informal re-check. Otherwise, the patient/athlete does not have regular contact with the team physician, and many times has limited contact with health care personnel. With this in mind, it becomes very important that attending health care personnel keep careful attention and regular contact with injured athletes to monitor their condition.

Likewise, because of insurance limitations, the patient/athlete will at best be seen for treatment only once per day and usually for a specified time (for example, 1 hour). Strict rules govern the level of care this person can receive. This includes the number of visits, the frequency in days per week, and the length in weeks for treatment. Rules will vary from insurer to insurer as well. It is best that the patient/athlete or athletic trainer/direct health care provider be familiar with insurance coverage, assuring that rehabilitative services are covered and to what extent their coverage extends. This will require familiarization by the team athletic trainer (or health care provider) with a variety of insurance companies and a brief understanding of their rules governing rehabilitation. These rules include maximum number of visits (often in a calendar year), denied services (such as "experimental" treatments), proper International Classification of Disease (ICD)-9 and Current Procedural Terminology (CPT) codes, and accurate documentation needed for reimbursement. Furthermore, the person providing care to the patient/athlete must do so under appropriate state statutes. In some cases, the team physician may have to coordinate care with the team athletic trainer in conjunction with other supervisory staff. This must be arranged and understood to insure a clear delegation of responsibilities to those persons caring for the athlete.

All of this is authorized through the physician prescription, which must be updated and signed regularly. It is also advisable that pre-authorization for treatment is obtained by the patient/athlete before initiating care, and that any paperwork such as incident reports and patient data be promptly filled out. Standing orders to provide care are rare in this setting, unlike those in a collegiate, university, or professional training room, and usually everything is governed by the physician prescription.

When setting up a team physician relationship with a health care provider in a clinical setting, it is advisable to establish a "standards of care" with the provider and the clinic. In this, there should be a general understanding of the level of care the patient/athlete will receive, and recognition that the in-clinic health care provider who is also associated with the team (often as the team's athletic trainer) will be coordinating and supervising the care of the patient/athlete. Communication is essential to establishing and maintaining this level of care, particularly when direct physician contact is limited.

An open understanding must be established between the physician's office and office staff and that of the clinic providing health care services to the patient/athlete. Communication between the team physician and the health care provider, such as that team's athletic trainer, should be open and immediate. If a problem occurs or there is a change in clinical findings, each person should be able to easily contact the other and work together to optimize the clinical outcome of the patient/athlete. This takes planning and protocols should be set up as the team physician and athletic trainer enter the season.

The team's athletic trainer or physical therapist usually coordinates most decision activities in the clinic setting regarding the patient/athlete, particularly when rehabilitative treatment is limited to once daily or once every other day (or less). The trainer or therapist supervises and oversees care and is duty-bound to insure that the injured athlete get the best care available. This care should be one-on-one between the health care provider associated with the team (team athletic trainer) and patient/athlete, with ancillary staff providing support. With this in mind, effective communication with the clinical health care provider and team physician is crucial to share important information such as MRI or radiographic findings, blood tests, or findings from specialists.

An effective scenario revolving around an injured athlete might present itself as follows:

The athlete is injured and evaluated on site by the health care provider (for example an athletic trainer at the high school). This initial visit is documented by the athletic trainer. The athlete is then referred to the team physician for further evaluation. The team physician sees the athlete either at the team's training room (best option) or later that day or the next, at the physician's office.

The athlete is evaluated by the team physician and referred, with prescription, to the rehabilitation clinic where the team's athletic trainer is employed. The injured athlete effectively becomes a patient, or patient/athlete. There, he or she is evaluated by the appropriate person. Depending on state law, this could be the athletic trainer or physical therapist. Treatment is initiated and additional in-clinic rehabilitation visits are scheduled. A home program is established and follow-up checks at the school or sports athletic training room are set.

An initial visit note is sent to the team physician describing the visit, establishing goals, and developing a treatment program. Subsequent treatment visits are properly documented in the patient/athlete's chart. If there are any abrupt changes in the health status of the patient/athlete, the team physician is contacted immediately.

Periodically, the patient/athlete is seen by the team physician. This can occur at either the rehabilitation clinic, the team's athletic training facility, or the physician's office. Progress is documented and adjustments to the treatment plan are formulated. Communications with the attending health care provider delivering care and team physician are conducted regularly either in writing, by phone, or in person at the team's training room or athletic facility.

Ideally, as the patient/athlete progresses in recovery, the attending health care provider will advance the exercise program, introducing sport-specific, functional exercises to prepare for return to participation. The team physician should be updated on this progress and the patient/athlete should be re-evaluated before any return-to-participation decisions are made. The team physician is obligated to be in the return-to-play decision-making, and as such must be in communication with the attending health care provider.

When working with clinical staff caring for athletes, the key task as a team physician is to establish open two-way communication between that staff person and the team physician. The purpose is to keep everyone working together to provide the proper care for the patient/athlete and allow return to participation as soon and safely as possible. All communication, in-clinic visits, and training room consultations and treatments should be properly documented in accordance with state and federal laws.

Working as a team physician associated with a clinical outreach program or athletic team attended to by clinic staff has numerous rewards. It enhances professional relationships and can help develop additional referral sources. If you, as a physician, are pleased with the care the patient/athlete receives, this particular clinic may be a good facility for the referral of other patients. Likewise, this clinic may become a site that will refer patients other than athletes to this team physician. Because of enhanced communication, clinic staff may be a good resource for answers to questions regarding specific rehabilitation concerns. And the clinical staff member you are working with in the care of a particular team or sport may become a friend and colleague. That is a good thing.

PROFESSIONAL SPORTS

The organizational structure of the professional team's medical staff has the same essential element of many high school and collegiate teams: the bond between the athletic training staff and the team physician. Obviously, many significant differences exist between what is expected at the pro team level and the high school or college levels, but the medical staff's bedrock foundation is the relationship of these professionals "in the trenches." Successful athletic trainer/ team physician duos are each other's staunchest advocates, in a relationship forged by respect and close friendship. Many times we providers are the bearers of bad news or see players at their lowest career phases because of injuries. On the other hand, we gladly take the back seat in sharing successes of players who rebound from an assortment of medical challenges.

There are many components to the medical staff of a professional team. Typically the head athletic trainer is comparable to the hub of a wheel, with the wheel's spokes representing all of the physicians and allied health consultants that make up the medical staff. In some cases the team's medical director is an orthopedic specialist, in others not. Regardless of their defined role, the orthopedic specialist and primary care provider are the most vital members of the medical staff. These two specialists will see virtually every injury that comes through the athletic training room, and make the appropriate recommendations and decisions. The goal is to keep things in-house and stay with the team physicians as much as possible. If a particular consultant needs to be involved, it will be the team physician who makes that suggestion. The orthopedic injury may require a subspecialist for the foot, hand, spine, or the like. Medical specialists will be consulted as the need arises. These may include physicians from the specialties of, but not limited to: internal medicine, ophthalmology, neurology, dermatology, cardiology, and dentistry. A women's team is likely to have a specialist in obstetrics/gynecology as a liaison. In many cases these physicians will attend games or be on somewhat of an on-call basis. Allied health consultants who are involved with a professional team may include physical therapists, chiropractors, and massage therapists. Again these consultants may attend games to provide their services as needed, or will be available on a more scheduled basis, such as at practices.

Other important pieces of the medical staff mosaic are laboratory and imaging services. It is not often that a player will need laboratory work, but the timing of the results is critical. As a result, most laboratory tests are considered "stat" in nature. As simple as it may seem, the choice of prescription medication may depend on laboratory results. The faster the results are back, the better it is for everyone. On- site radiographs are required, recommended, or at least suggested for professional sports venues. Many times the convenience of radiographs at the arena or stadium makes life easier for the physician and athlete. The radiographs are read by the team's medical staff on site; thus it is not be likely that a radiologist will be present. There will be many radiological needs and the results of these are "stat" also. Imaging such as MRI, CT scan, or bone scan all seem to be ordered routinely, or certainly much more frequently than in the non-athletic world. Centers that provide these services generally accommodate the player's schedule as much as possible to expedite the examination. Once the image is complete, the radiologist will provide a report to the team physician for conveyance to the athletic trainer. Last, but certainly not least, the final elements of a typical medical staff for a professional team are the emergency personnel. As first responders, athletic trainers are trained in cardiopulmonary resuscitation (CPR) and automated external defibrillator (AED) use. Also, all have a structured plan for an emergency situation for the day-to-day practices, off days, off-season, and other periods. The coverage for game days will vary based on the potential of an emergency in the sport. Basketball or baseball may have an on-site ambulance, paramedics, and emergency medical technicians. If there is one rule of thumb, it is that the emergency medical staff should stay at a game venue until the players have left the premises. Football requires a physician on the sidelines who is skilled in intubation, in addition to ambulance and emergency medical personnel.

What has been described up until now is the routine day-to-day process when the team is at home. It's important to keep in mind that half of the professional team's games are away, which presents an occasional medical challenge. In football, the team's physicians travel with the team; thus their routine seems to change the least. In the other sports, the athletic trainer relies on the host team's physicians as needed. Routinely, the athletic trainer will stay in touch with his team physician while traveling. This contact will consist of simple updates or status reports, as well as relating information on a new injury. If needed, the host team's athletic trainer will go out of his way to help. This assistance could be evaluating a player injury that occurred during a game, or setting up diagnostic tests that the team physician has called in from home. It is common practice for a host physician to also call the team's physician when the team relies on him to evaluate or treat an injury. This professionalism and camaraderie is very important within the ranks of both the athletic trainers and team physicians.

The head athletic trainer and team physician are the medical voices that speak to the players, coaching staff, and team management. In many cases, members of the coaching staff or team management will meet with the medical staff in a regular and casual manner. This informal conversational type of meeting maintains a good information flow. More formal reporting methods and styles may vary with the individual team. Ultimately, team management does know how to get the information it needs. As specialists or consultants diagnose injuries, it will be the team physician who condenses the information for explanation to the team. Thus accurate communication between all parties involved is vital.

One element that is somewhat unique at the pro team level compared with the high school or college level is the interaction with the media. Communication with the local or national media is part of the daily world of professional sports. It is important for all people involved in the public dissemination of a player's medical information to convey the same message, in the same manner, at the same time. This minimizes confusion, prevents rumors from circulating, and most importantly, respects the player's privacy. To keep the medical information accurate, the team physician or athletic trainer may discuss the injury status with the player, coaching staff, and management to determine the extent of information to be made public. That information can then be conveyed to the team's media relations department for distribution to the media. This policy protects the player's privacy and is not an attempt at "one-upmanship" or hiding information, while respecting the public's interest.

Care and caution should be exercised in cases when the medical staff addresses the media directly. Some teams opt to have their medical staff address the media on a routine basis. For teams that route this information through the media relations personnel, the team physician or athletic trainer might address the media if an injury or its care is complicated. The purpose may be to address generalities of the case or translate medical information into lay terms. No matter what the circumstances, it is vitally important to include the player's input on information provided to the media.

At times, managing the professional athlete's medical care is straightforward: player sustains an injury, reports it to the athletic training staff, and it is referred to the team physician for the appropriate disposition. On the other hand, there are instances in which the medical staff needs to work cooperatively with layers of well-wishers and personal advocates in the player's camp. These may include family members, friends, business associates, and the player's agent.

When the player advocates involve themselves in medical care, it is important for everyone to sustain a professional level of communication and cooperation. It is quite possible that an agent will seek a second opinion in a surgical situation. This opinion might come from a physician that the agent has had a longstanding relationship with. If the physician is credible in sports medicine, it can be a win-win situation for all involved. Either way, it is important that the team physician and the outside consultant discuss the case with the player's best interest in mind. Despite the way things "should" be managed, there will be times that a player will take medical matters into his own hands and seek his own physician without the team or agent knowing about it. This case catches everyone by surprise. In that situation, the hope is that the player's concerns and team's goals still mesh together.

Being a team physician for a professional team might be the second most exciting job in sports medicine, only behind being the athletic trainer for a pro team. If a successful team physician's characteristics were profiled, being a sports fan would be very high on the list. Some team physicians have been collegiate athletes and others have been Olympic or professional athletes. Many have membership in the National Athletic Trainers Association, American College of Sports Medicine, or a professional society such as the American Orthopedic Society for Sports Medicine. This role at the professional team level demands a tremendous amount of personal and professional time. Obviously, the game and team practice schedules have their needs, but also it is the non-business hours that can cut into family time. The range of this time demand could go from a phone call in the middle of the night to a playoff game on the road on the same day as a wedding anniversary. It all goes with the territory.

As previously noted, the team's medical landscape will include a variety of consultants and second opinion providers. A value of a skilled team physician is to have the best local specialists to consult on a player's situation, seemingly at a moment's notice. The network of physicians at the fingertips of the team physician is very important. If an outside consultant is called in, the team physician needs the player examined as quickly as possible to establish a diagnosis and plan of care. The team may need to make personnel decisions based on the medical information. A strength of a skilled team physician is to know when to defer to the specialist or outside opinion, while maintaining the role as the team's advocate for the player's care. Maybe the strongest suit of a successful team physician at the professional team level is good old-fashioned bedside manner. Professional athletes rely on the well-being of their bodies to provide income. The team is as strong as its weakest link. When an injury or illness compromises any player's ability, it is very comforting for all involved to know that the team physician is a friend, advocate, and caring professional.

OLYMPIC SPORTS MEDICINE FOR THE TEAM PHYSICIAN

The Olympic dream, at its very essence, is founded on the ideal that athleticism, in purest form, is defined by total commitment to attain peak performance timed precisely during world competition. Sportsmanship and fair play underscore the competitive experience as the "best of the best" display skill, preparation, and dedication epitomizing pushing the limits to succeed. As a result of this inherent intensity, Olympic competition creates an environment for significant injury.

Team physician designation for an international sporting event is both exhilarating and intimidating in equal doses. Appropriate medical coverage at an Olympic venue poses a challenging mandate to provide state-of-the-art sports medicine care to a unique group of elite world class athletes. In addition to a wide variety of sports-specific musculoskeletal injuries, the Olympic venue physician must be prepared to treat potentially serious medical emergencies. Prior interscholastic, collegiate, and professional sports game day coverage experience provides the foundation for emergency evaluation and time-sensitive medical decision-making.

Olympic Venue Physician Selection Process

Selection as an Olympic physician begins with investigation of volunteer opportunities at one of the Olympic training centers, followed by assignments at United States Olympic Committee (USOC)-sponsored events with positive evaluative performances. Injured athlete care at the Olympic training center parallels the design at the high school or college level, with a team of athletic trainers and support staff dedicated to on going care. Conversely, medical attention to elite athletes at an international event affords a different experience. The clinical significance of a complaint must be assessed under field conditions and the intensity of world-class competition, away from one's customary staff, equipment, and facilities. Further, this is done with limited previous knowledge of the athlete and with the assistance of a new team of sports medicine professionals working together. Colleagues with prior involvement in Olympic events or national team coverage provide an excellent resource for clinical advice and insight to the international aspects of sports medicine delivery, in addition to networking for future opportunities.

Olympic Venue Regulations: Assessing the Environment

The Olympic venue athlete experience is designed to afford fair play and strict control of the competitive event. On the day of participation athletes will transition from the warm-up area, with access to both the venue medical staff and individual international medical teams, to the competition venue 30 minutes before participation. After competing, athletes exit the field of play and enter the "mixed zone" to initiate post-event testing and potential medical attention. Organizing committee staff, security personal, and drug testing officials all have defined responsibilities in this zone. The location for credentialed press is usually adjacent to the mixed zone entry. The athlete medical care clinic is typically located in close proximity. Depending on the venue, national team physicians may have athlete access.

The Olympic venue sports medicine team is responsible for evaluating injuries occurring in each of these areas. Each site is unique in its environment and regulations governing decision-making in a timely fashion. To avoid confusion and potential chaotic situations, the Olympic team physician must exercise leadership by providing clarity in the differential diagnosis and injury management options. Skillful athletic trainer resource use during elite athlete competition is essential.

Team Physician and Athletic Trainer Teamwork

The lead athletic trainer typically serves as the liaison between the medical staff and the related event personnel and necessary local services. The coordination of services and timing of delivery become paramount in the planning process.

Special consideration must be given to the specific event and to what potential catastrophes exist. The carefully evaluated physical aspects of the event facility and local geography play an important role in the equipment and transportation needs on-site. This requires the development of potential scenarios and trial runs of treatment plans from on-site care to emergency room delivery to assess efficacy. This "scrimmage" experience provides valuable information to determine specific equipment needs, number of staff required, and route mapping.

During the development of emergency planning the lead team should concurrently compile the competencies required of the staff members. Team physician-designed protocols, with any specific language code words, should be used commonly by all members of the medical team to avoid confusion. The staff should be assembled in advance of the event to review the "protocol playbook," assemble specific response teams, and practice with equipment to be used.

The collaborative development of the team physician and athletic trainer relationship relies on communication. The specific skills of both professionals are vital to provide accurate assessment and treatment in a potentially stressful situation. The careful pre-event planning, scrimmaging, and protocol development provide the learning curve in regards to the assignment of duties. The specialties of each lead team member should be clear, and this information should be used as the staffing needs are considered.

Olympic Venue Athlete Medical Care: Warm-up Facility

Warm-up facilities provide a venue for athletes to prepare for an upcoming event. When separate warm-up facilities, which may be at a separate location, are provided, all logistical considerations must be made in the same fashion as the competitive venue. A separate staff will be necessary, but all protocols and equipment considerations should be the same for both areas to allow for staff exchange between the two sites. Facility evaluation, emergency, and transportation issues warrant the same attention to detail as the competitive venue.

The warm-up facility differs significantly from the field of play in that athletes will have direct contact with their delegation cohort, and most athletes will have a support staff to provide routine treatment and physical preparation for competition. In some cases, athletes will arrive without a support staff. This requires the development of a treatment area and staff for therapeutic purposes in addition to emergency care. The design of this area will usually be affected by the space available, but should include at a minimum the modalities to treat the most common injuries sustained by the athletes in the specific event of the site. The planning process should include the ability to treat acute as well as chronic musculoskeletal conditions.

Staffing the warm-up venue also requires the same considerations as the field-of-play venue. The lead team must consider the volume of athletes, the schedule of specific events, and the risk of catastrophic injury involved with the specific sport in order to effectively fill staff requirements. On-site emergency care and orthopedic physicians, along with athletic trainers and paramedic-trained emergency medical services (EMS) personnel, should be a minimum requirement. Other disciplines should be considered, because many athletes will request spinal manipulation, massage therapy, and other non-acute treatments.

Olympic Venue Athlete Medical Care: Field-of-Play Priorities

Priorities on the field of play ultimately sort out the expedient and efficient response to trauma sustained by athletes. As described, the planning and scrimmage process before the actual event is paramount to the successful delivery of care. Priority goes to potential catastrophic and life-threatening trauma. This requires careful consideration of the environment as well as the specific event. Every effort should be made to forecast the potential for chaotic situations that may involve multiple individuals, such as endurance events in weather extremes, or a collision leaving two or more injured or unconscious athletes.

Communication deserves careful consideration. The lead team should have direct communication with staff on the field of play, attending EMS personnel, on-site treatment area, and local emergency department. Staff should have the opportunity to practice with radio equipment, and a communication specialist should be a part of the medical team to ensure that equipment is maintained and functioning properly at all times.

Priority equipment includes devices that provide the most accurate vital sign data in an expedient fashion, and that can be easily transported with the victim to the on-site treatment area or local trauma facility. Portable vital sign devices that provide blood pressure, temperature, oxygen saturation, and pulse allow trending-based treatment and decisions to occur accurately and expediently. In addition, advanced cardiac life support (ACLS) equipment and pharmacology supplies should be readily available and strategically placed based on where vulnerable events take place. This equipment should be compatible with local emergency services, including EMS and local emergency departments.

After lifesaving equipment is considered, immobilization devices, including spine board and c-spine management, and fracture care must be considered. Special attention must be given to the specific equipment worn in sport as well. All decisions regarding the management of protective equipment should be evaluated with regard to removal and specific tools that may be needed. It is standard practice to rehearse any potential situation with the actual equipment.

Bodily fluids pose a specific risk in athletics. Universal precautions, treatment of blood-related injury, and the rules governing the specific sport pose a challenge in several circumstances. It is important to review the rules of the specific sport governing the effect of open wounds. Some sports, such as wrestling, impose time limits in which the bleeding must stopped before the risk of forfeiture. Most sports will require the athlete to leave the field of play when bleeding occurs and don a clean uniform before return. The medical staff usually play a significant role in this process, and may impact the event if not properly prepared.

Olympic Venue Athlete Medical Care: Mixed-Zone Triage

Medical triage for athletes in the mixed zone requires careful selection of sports medicine personal with event-specific experience and keen sports trauma-evaluation skills to provide injury screening in this often chaotic setting. Language barriers, post-event anxiety with patriotic failure perceptions, and previous injury complaints pose formidable obstacles to stratifying the degree of injury. Bottled water and sports drink, all sealed, are available for initial treatment of heat illness, with strict instructions for the athlete to choose from a cooler to avoid controversy in subsequent drug testing. The decision to transport the athlete to the athlete care clinic for a more comprehensive evaluation may include input from the medical team from his or her country, with or without availability of a translator. The mixed-zone staff typically defers vital sign assessment and relies on directed physical examinations for injury grading.

Olympic Venue Athlete Medical Care: Athlete Medical Clinic

The athlete care medical station is typically located close to the competition exit and serves as command center for coordination of all components of injury management once athletes enter the warm-up training location on the day of competing. Registration and record keeping are mandated priorities and require a significant expenditure of time and talent.

Strains and sprains are the most common injuries encountered in Olympic athletes. The injury evaluation and treatment area with standard modalities requires the largest space in the athlete care clinic. In addition to new complaints, many athletes will have pre-existing musculoskeletal conditions and require continuity of prior care rendered. Therapeutic interventions of all kinds need to be available.

The medical sport trauma area needs a minimum of two dedicated beds with vital sign monitoring, intravenous fluids, and airway support. Trauma bed design must facilitate prompt evaluation in cases of heat stress, cardiopulmonary emergencies, and head and neck injury. Each bed should be budgeted space for a three- to five-member treatment team. In the case of head and neck emergencies, standard treatment initiated on the field of play needs to be continuous, providing seamless transition during transport and trauma bed.

Sports Trauma Preparation

The Olympic team physician has responsibility for providing leadership for both the initial evaluation of a variety of routine and expected orthopedic injuries, as well as the less frequent and unexpected cases of serious medical sports trauma. Elite athlete collapse during strenuous participation is uncommon, and in the case of endurance events is usually related to post-event fatigue; however, initial evaluation of the downed athlete needs a high index of suspicion for potential head, heart, heat, or respiratory compromise.

The trauma room requires expert preparation in floor design, team member tasking, and equipment use. Physician supervision and attention to detail is essential for successful emergency management protocol design. Four- or five-member teams should be assigned to each trauma suite, with an additional floor marking for an interpreter. Each room should be equipped with all standard ACLS equipment and supplies. The physician leader should be ideally positioned next to cardiac monitor/defibrillator on the patient's right side, with initial and serial vital sign assessment obtained and recorded on a trauma board on the opposite side of the bed. The head of position requires skills in airway issues and head and neck injury management. The fourth team member at the foot of the bed must have communication capabilities to coordinate care with national team physicians as well as venue medical command, while also providing crowd control.

Whenever possible, a preliminary venue visit affords a calculated and expert design to use budgeted medical service space and facilities. Sport trauma bed design with existing treatment protocol can then be tested in a local setting with familiar staff at a sports clinic or emergency department, simulating venue conditions with mock patients.

Initial vital sign assessment in the context of the reported injury mechanism and venue conditions guide early differential diagnosis decisions and severity of trauma grading. Vital sign trending recorded at 5-minute intervals on the Olympic venue athlete trauma board provide the basic information required to monitor treatment response and document the need for transport to the assigned hospital emergency department. Vital sign trending should continue for 30 minutes. Return-to-competition decisions remain a priority during this initial evaluation. Athletes who have a subjective improvement combined with return-to-baseline vital signs are candidates for continued participation. Persistent tachycardia in this group of well-conditioned athletes is of special concern, and requires additional monitoring and 12-lead EKG assessments.

Heat Stress and Asthma Protocols

Emergency care for heat stress and asthma requires a high priority of preparedness at mass gatherings displaying high-intensity athleticism from a wide variety of climates and air environments. Most world competitions are scheduled at the high and low ends of predicted regional temperatures to afford the best conditions for competition. Travel requirements may not allow adequate time for optimal acclimatization. Environmental allergens and air quality vary greatly among participating nations. Dry conditions are planned for summer competition, and cold weather for winter sports. As a result, both extremes provide triggers for exercise-induced asthma precipitated by cold, dry conditions.

Heightened awareness of the syndrome of exercise-induced asthma in elite athletes occurred in conjunction with the 1984 Summer Olympic Games in Los Angeles. After observing a significant occurrence of respiratory difficulties during the 1984 winter games in Sarajevo, the US Olympic Training Center conducted a screening program to identify athletes at risk. Eleven point two per cent of summer game athletes were discovered to have exercise-induced asthma (67 of a total of 597 athletes screened).

Sometimes termed "the hidden syndrome," respiratory compromise without a history of prior diagnosis may be present in world class athletes during or after competition. Accurate diagnosis of exercise-induced asthma in this group of elite athletes presents a challenge to the Olympic sports medicine team. All athletes reporting breathing difficulties or unusual shortness of breath should be carefully assessed using rehearsed protocols (Table 2).

Athletes with documentation of the syndrome are readily identified through event medical records and the onset of wheezing or post-event coughing.

Athletes who have respiratory compromise need prompt evaluation with monitored vital signs, including cardiac monitoring and continuous oxygen saturation. Tympanic measurements for temperature are preferred secondary to rapid respiratory rates. The peak expiratory flow meter initial measurement is extremely helpful in rapidly determining the severity of bronchoconstriction. If available, end-tidal CO_2 capnography assessment may be helpful in severe cases.

Heat Stress

Heat stress is a common medical condition in summer competitions. High temperature, humidity, and radiant heating in host countries, combined with altered perceived exertion limits in international competition, result in increased rates of heat emergencies among athletes. Since the 1992 Barcelona Games, where temperatures reached the low 90s, continuous venue climatic measurements of dry bulb temperature (DBT), wet bulb temperature (WBT), and black bulb temperature have become the standard in providing

Table 2
Asthma protocol 1996 Atlanta Games Olympic Stadium

Place athletes in sports trauma bed 1 or 2	Three-member team optimal
Oxygen saturation monitor with complete vital signs (record on trauma board)	Consider cardiac monitor if severe symptoms, except O2 sat >95%
Peak flow measurement and record	PEFR <300 L/min severe, consider end tidal CO2
Offer O2 face mask NRB@10 L/min	If apprehensive with mask, consider hand-held instead of strapped
Offer albuterol MDI, two puffs	
If no improvement in 10 minutes, repeat vital signs and nebulizer Rx	Consider nebulized treatment if no prior inhaler use
Repeat peak flow meter at 15 minutes	If PEFR returns to predicted baseline, consider return to competition

Abbreviations: NRB, non–re-breather mask; PEFR, peak flow.

medical personal valuable information for accurate heat stress index calculations. The climatic heat stress index (HIS) temperature is calculated by combining 70% of the WBT and 10% of the DBT readings. In preparation for the 1996 Atlanta Olympic Games, pre-event research by Dr. David Martin from Georgia State University resulted in a change in the men's marathon time from 6:30 PM, coordinated with closing ceremonies, to 7:00 AM to minimize heat stress. This change was prompted after a 3-year investigation into temperature trends in Atlanta during late July and early August.

Heat stress in the Olympic environment typically presents as post-event weakness with mild dehydration. Heat exhaustion is less frequent, and initial vital signs typically reveal mild temperature elevations and pulse rates above 100. Heat stroke with cardiovascular collapse is rare, and the finding of persistent temperature elevation and hypotension requires rapid cooling and emergency transport for hospital admission and laboratory support. Athletes who have suspected heat stress during competition require prompt evaluation in the venue medical clinic. A 30-minute period of observation with rehearsed protocol will provide valuable information, allowing athlete stratification in a timely fashion. The heat illness protocol used at Olympic Stadium for track and field and marathon competition during the 1996 Atlanta Games is listed in Table 3 for reference. Real time climatic conditions from venue staff provide "high index of suspicion" time frames for athletes during warm-up, competition, and post event mixed-zone evaluations.

The use of intravenous fluid for dehydration, although mandatory for inability to tolerate oral hydration, remains an attractive treatment modality for accelerated recovery with vital sign normalization. Triathletes and other same-day multi-event participants during high heat index periods are candidates for isotonic normal saline fluid therapy. In addition to documentation of

---

Table 3
Heat illness: post-event weakness protocol 1996 Atlanta Games Olympic Stadium

	Clinical guidelines for management
1. Place athlete on trauma bed 1 or 2.	Oral or tympanic temperatures unless unconscious with rectal measurements
2. Record initial VS on trauma board.	
3. If pulse >140, BP <100 systolic, or O2 Sat <90, place on cardiac monitor and face mask at 10 L/min and IV NS bolus.	Expect mild tachycardia with normal to high BP
	Nausea suggests heat exhaustion with need for IV
4. Offer cold water 500 cc.	Transport criteria: altered mental status, seizure, persistent temp elevation
5. Ice-water towel on groin, axilla, and neck	
6. Consider IV after 15 minutes of cooling; oral fluids not tolerated.	Discharge criteria: VS normalization, not orthostatic, tolerating oral fluids
7. Repeat vital every 5 minutes and record.	
8. Rectal probe temp if oral temp >102 at 10 minutes.	

Abbreviations: BP, blood pressure; NS, normal saline; VS, vital sign.

a normal temperature, return-to-play criteria for elite athletes who have heat stress requires the absence of tachycardia and a negative assessment of postural hypotension.

The Olympic Experience

The selection as an Olympic team physician is a career milestone and provides a once-in-a-lifetime experience to showcase talent and dedication to the discipline of sports medicine. Diligent preparation and focus is required to maximize this opportunity. Early contact with the venue medical director and athletic trainer will facilitate knowledge of planned medical facilities and equipment. An on-site visit before competition affords an opportunity to review and modify proposed protocols for sports trauma management. Finally, and perhaps most important, the Olympic experience should be a shared event with family members. Their support and the memories generated will result in a patriotic celebration to be shared for generations.

Acknowledgments

The authors thank Dr. Del Bolin for critical reading of the manuscript.

Reference

[1] Stockard AR. Team physician preferences at National Collegiate Athletic Association Division I universities. J Am Osteopath Assoc 1997;2:89–95.

Clin Sports Med 26 (2007) 227–241

CLINICS IN SPORTS MEDICINE

SEVIER
JNDERS

Financial Implications of Serving as Team Physician

Larry Lemak, MD

Alabama Sports Medicine and Orthopaedic Center, 806 St. Vincent's Drive, Suite 415, Birmingham, AL 35205, USA

This article discusses the financial aspects of being a team physician. As you will read, the dollars and cents play a small role in the actual decision-making process in a contractual relationship between a team physician and an organization. Effective and successful contractual arrangements require experience, diplomatic skills, and a strong understanding of one's time and worth. It is not uncommon to see a team physician's role undergo change with an organization as a result of the many intangibles associated with the overall arrangement.

Although it is very important to completely understand the financial aspects of being a team physician, it should not be the driving force behind one's decision to serve in such a role. When we talk about the financial implications, an old saying comes to mind: "Is it about the money? It's always about the money." If this were not true, you would not see the level of competition for jobs as a team physician, regardless of the level of play. There is no question that being a team physician can be an important financial component to your practice.

As is discussed below, however, know that serving as a team physician, like all other professional choices that one will make, can be both a positive and negative experience. This is dictated by the ability to plan and organize predictable financial implications related to the investment put into the role.

Financial reimbursement does not only appear in the form of a designated dollar agreement, because additional methods of compensation and or satisfaction may be seen as benefits of serving as a team physician. The actual cost of your time when you are standing on the sidelines of events, traveling, or simply visiting the training rooms of the teams that you cover can be very high. This is not only time away from your medical practice, but it also is time away from your family and personal life. Expectations for your services as a team physician tend to be 24 hours a day, 7 days a week regardless of what contractual arrangement you may have or the level of competition you are providing

E-mail address: jkonin@health.usf.edu

0278-5919/07/$ – see front matter
doi:10.1016/j.csm.2007.01.003 © 2007 Published by Elsevier Inc.
sportsmed.theclinics.com

services for. In sports, every injury to every athlete is the most important at any given time!

Common circumstances can lead to many indirect adverse financial considerations. For example, "VIP" treatment of athletes who want immediate accessibility will lead to impromptu interruptions, and thus require you to take time away from your scheduled patients and other preplanned events. This will also have an impact on your office staff, unexpectedly taking up more of their time. Accessibility and timely evaluations and treatments are the minimal expectation coaches and players have of a team physician at any level of sport, yet among the most difficult items to attach a financial worth to.

Some who have served in the role of a team physician in the past have informally talked about what is referred to as "charity" work, or treating uninsured athletes. This reality holds true especially at the high school and college levels, where your title as team physician places you in an expected position to treat everyone regardless of the insurance or lack thereof.

Some of the financial considerations will be determined by the level of competition that you may be providing care for. Significant differences exist among high school, college, professional, Olympic, and other levels of sports. To further complicate this matrix of comparison, there is so much variation from sport to sport that serving as a team physician will lead you to question which aspects, levels, and sports are worth your valuable time. Higher levels of competition bring additional necessary travel, along with possible increased pre- and postseason obligations. All of these expected commitments must be factored into the equation when evaluating the finances of being a team physician.

There is very little about this subject in our professional literature to rely on or refer to for advice. I rely heavily on my personal experience of being a team physician for 30 years at all levels of competition. I have also found that collaboration with experienced team physicians and friends can be most helpful. Though it is difficult to put a dollar figure on such intangibles as personal satisfaction, ego, and stature in the local and national communities as a result of being a high-profile team physician, unquestionably these have clear and very high value.

FORMS OF CONTRACTUAL ARRANGEMENTS

In general, there are four ways to serve in a relationship as a team physician that have financial implications related to your services. Two of these methods include a documented exchange of money, either from the organization to the team physician, or from the team physician to the organization. One method does not involve actual cash exchange, but rather soft-money exchange in the form of various intangibles. Lastly, serving in a volunteer capacity does not involve a formal exchange or contractual agreement, yet it does have financial implications.

Fee for Service

A fee-for-service contractual arrangement is perhaps the most basic contractual type. In the agreement, the physician receives a prearranged sum of money on a fixed-term basis for prearranged, agreed-on services to be provided in return. The fixed-term could be anywhere from months to years, with incremental changes and criteria to be met for continued services. The prearranged services can include on-site coverage and care for a certain number of days or games, commitments to evaluate acute injuries within a given period of time, costs of certain types of imaging and procedures in a limited or capitated manner, medical supplies, and many other reasonable, ethical, and legal negotiable services.

Advantages of fee for service
The clear advantage associated with a fee-for-service contract is the ability to prognosticate one's financial future in exchange for the time and service commitment; however, as we all know, health care changes rapidly, and some forms of fixed financial arrangements may fluctuate in an ongoing manner. Furthermore, there is no doubt that an experienced team physician who has analyzed previous years of financial exchanges in such a role will have a keener awareness of attaching a dollar figure to all fixed agreements.

Disadvantages of fee for service
The clear disadvantage of establishing a fixed fee-for-service arrangement stems from the inexperience of the team physician with predicting the total service needed by a given team or organization for the length of the contract. This again relates to the inexperience or unfamiliarity with being a team physician as it relates to the overall management of the business aspect of the services required for a particular team or organization. Accurate analysis is critical, because if a physician overcharges, then the organization's administration will pay careful attention to this and use it for bargaining power for future negotiations. If one undercharges, it makes for a more difficult renegotiation when asking for an increase in dollars. This can be used as a reason for an organization to make a change with service providers and avoid a negotiation process.

Paying to Serve as Team Physician
There are occasions where physicians or the business that they are associated with will pay for the rights to serve as the official team physicians for a certain organization. This is seen more commonly with high- profile sports that receive greater national exposure, such as professional teams or major level (Division I) colleges and universities. The main reason for such a relationship is for the reservation of rights, which indirectly would exclude others from having the same privilege. In some cases, a university that operates publicly and does not have physicians employed as permanent faculty or staff must contract externally to the physician or physician group that provides the best offer. In such cases, "best" is oftentimes determined by the committee conducting the search for the institution, and along with the experience, quality of care, and accessibility that can be provided by a physician, financial arrangements are an important aspect of the evaluative process.

The issue of actually paying to become a team physician is hotly debated these days. Because of the competitive nature of our business and profession, the ethical issues must be dealt with regarding this topic, perhaps more so than any other administrative aspect of the role and responsibility of being a team physician. There is a lot at stake financially in becoming a team physician, and ethical guidelines must not be overlooked.

Advantages of paying to serve as team physician
The single main reason for paying to serve as a team physician revolves around holding exclusive rights to the services and using such rights for marketing advantages. Using television and radio broadcasts, stationary, and other media outlets to convey the message that you are the official provider for a sought-after organization has significant market value that is difficult to accurately measure financially. Furthermore, it lends itself to perceived automatic credibility by members of the general public, who identify you in the role as the chosen provider of services to that important organization, therefore causing them to seek your care as well.

Disadvantages of paying to serve as team physician
The major objective disadvantage of actually paying as a physician for the rights to provide your services is seen in the expenses associated with the contractual agreement. All other tangible items such as time and services may not be any different in terms of a commitment. Within the medical profession, many see this type of an arrangement as being unethical, strictly because the decision to hire a team physician is not based on qualifications but instead solely on financial terms. Though contractual agreements are confidential, it is not difficult to determine if a provider is paying or being paid to serve in the role of team physician. Providers who pay for the rights to serve as a team physician may quietly be perceived by others in a negative manner from an ethical perspective.

Soft-Money Arrangement
A contractual arrangement with no dollar value associated with it can be referred to as a "soft- money" arrangement. In this case, a physician or group agrees to provide team physician services without asking for a fee for service in return, and without buying the rights to serve as a team physician. One of the greatest benefits on the list of intangibles of serving as a team physician is job satisfaction and enjoyment. Individuals operating within a sole proprietorship who find the time and ability to serve as a team physician often do it for the love of their job and association with coaches, athletes, parents, and others affiliated with sports.

This can often be a changing landscape, however, and satisfaction can decrease over time. One team physician put this very well:

> My enjoyment level has diminished over the years. My first year involved with the team was the greatest thing ever. However, my enjoyment has waned over the years. The analogy I use taking care of a major league team is like dating the prettiest girl in your neighborhood growing up as a child. You felt fortunate that the prettiest girl in the neighborhood liked

you and that she would walk down the street holding your hand. However, she is now no longer quite that pretty and a pain in the neck, but you know as soon as you break up with her, she will date one of your friends. Therefore, one of the main reasons why I continue to take care of a major league team is that I do not want to give that advantage to any of my competitors. So, although she is a pain in the neck, she is my pain in the neck.
                                                                    —Anonymous

Many examples exist that could be considered in a negotiation of soft money in return for services; here are just a few:

- Complimentary tickets and parking passes
- Clothing and official attire
- Travel and accommodations for family
- Rights to being named as being formally affiliated through any dissemination of marketing information
- Advertisement in print and broadcast media
- Invitation as a guest to VIP events
- Access to facilities for usage of functions
- Vehicle mileage reimbursement
- Concessions coupons

Advantages of soft-money arrangement
Undoubtedly, the privilege and exclusive right to having a relationship with a team or organization brings with it many unpredictable benefits. For example, how much would you pay for an advertisement in a local or national newspaper? What part of the ad will justify your credibility and status? When you are mentioned in a newspaper article as the person taking care of an elite athlete, the credibility factor can be very powerful. This is of course assuming that the article is a positive one, and not about a failed surgery or rehabilitation of an athlete. Remember, members of the public can be very astute about name recognition, and often seek out the named team physician for their own care. Furthermore, television and print ads can be very costly. You will find that many of your patients come to see you and mention that they read about you in the newspaper or saw you on the sidelines of a game. Rarely do they mention that they saw your newspaper advertisement.

Disadvantages of soft-money arrangement
Although compensation by way of soft-money exchange can sometimes be immeasurable in terms of the indirect benefits that it can provide, keep in mind that the amount of compensation is not usually on par with one's normal compensation as a physician. Perhaps of most importance is that some will perceive this type of a relationship as being unethical in not receiving a fee for one's service. It is important to identify the details of the arrangement before jumping to conclusions. A physician may be well-qualified, semi-retired from private practice, and choose to give back time in this form, thereby not being unethical in terms of buying the rights to be the team physician. What organization would

not be excited about such an opportunity? Younger physicians are typically at a disadvantage in such a circumstance, because they may not have the time or money to donate. Furthermore, not having partnership status in a practice will limit one's ability to make such a choice.

Volunteering

When one volunteers services as a team physician there is no formal contractual arrangement and no expectations of services to be provided. Volunteer services are seen more often these days in smaller communities, where business competition is not of the highest intensity, and instead community building, in which most people know each other, takes precedence.

Advantages of volunteering

With volunteering comes less time commitment and clinical practice interruption, because any services that are provided are typically appreciated and not expected. Many team physicians will tell you that the role is indirectly accompanied by a varying level of stress that creeps its way into the job and rises and falls in an unpredictable manner. When you volunteer, you are not obligated under any circumstances to feel such pressures, because you can step aside at any time if you no longer enjoy the role. Furthermore, when you are volunteering in a small community where you truly know the people more personally, it is less likely that you will be treated as a business associate and more likely that such interpersonal relationships will reduce any unwanted stress that might otherwise come with the role. As discussed previously, any affiliation with a team or organization does bring with it many indirect perquisites by way of association.

Disadvantages of volunteering

Obviously a volunteer role brings with it no financial reward in return; however, it is questionable whether or not this can be seen as a disadvantage, because all who serve in this role clearly do so by choice. Perhaps three areas to be cautious with as they relate to a volunteer role are: (1) ambiguity, (2) overcommitment, and (3) liability. Not having a clearly defined role through a formalized contract can provide for some flexibility; however, it can also create some gray areas. In what capacity will you volunteer? Will there be some clinical conditions, procedures, and the like, that you won't feel comfortable dealing with in a volunteer role? These should at least be agreed upon early on, despite lack of a formal contract. There is an old saying that goes like this: "People who get things done right and in an efficient manner get rewarded with more work." Be careful not to continuously say "yes" to the point where your volunteer goals have risen higher than expected right before your eyes and have become the expected standard. Lastly, the non-clarity of having a formal agreement can truly add to circumstances whereby the role you play is uncertain to many. With uncertainty comes a much greater risk for opening oneself up to liability. Be sure that those you care for in a volunteer role clearly know what to expect and not to expect from you.

OVERALL COST CONSIDERATIONS

So many things are left to be considered when exploring the financial ramifications of serving as a team physician. Unless carefully planned out, each of these can be viewed as an adverse component of the relationship. By contrast, careful intuition can lead to a fruitful and long-lasting experience and relationship.

Perhaps one of the most expensive items needed to support your role as a team physician is the increased malpractice premiums you might pay when associated with a professional team. With risk and with valued investments, your margin for mistakes does not increase, but the magnification of your work does. Therefore, anyone unable to play who is being paid to perform may look askance at you for not making them better. Liability insurance at such a level is a must. Although not seen in increasing demands higher than normal elsewhere, one should not rule out the possibility of seeing higher premiums requested for anyone serving in a team physician role, despite the level of competition. More and more sudden deaths among youths have attracted national media attention, and may serve as the driving force behind such action.

The time commitment is extremely variable according to the level and type of sport. Previously agreed-upon expectations will also determine your total time commitment. Some of the responsibilities that may influence your time will be

- The need for preseason and exit physicals
- Coverage expectations
- Travel expectations
- VIP event expectations
- Number of total teams/athletes
- Length of seasons
- Sole or shared team physician responsibilities

In discussion with colleagues, one professional football team physician felt it took him 800 hours annually to provide appropriate coverage his team. This includes games, training room visits, training camp, National Football League (NFL) combines, minicamps, and physicals. This estimated figure did not even include any travel time. Another professional football team physician felt that he spent 100 days in some capacity or another providing coverage and care for his team. One professional soccer team physician felt that he spent 30 days a year taking care of the team. With professional baseball, there are 162 games and the normal expectation is to cover home games. There are also a total of 6 weeks of spring training camp. In baseball, you don't have the wear and tear of the travel schedule as a team physician, but in turn, you cover 81 games. The expected time spent at the home games is usually from a half hour before game time to a half hour after the game ends. Major league baseball games take anywhere from 3 to 4 hours, so the time spent during game nights can vary anywhere from a minimum of 3 hours up to 5 hours.

When you serve as a team physician for college sports, you are usually responsible for all sports, and must determine what the expectations of the school are regarding coverage of each sport and your ability to fulfill their needs. A college commitment can add up to 900 hours a year among all the different sports, including football, men and women's basketball, baseball, and soccer. There are very few standards here, although football coverage is expected because of the high injury rate seen. Other sports that are covered may be based on: (1) the risk of injury associated with the sport; (2) the geographical location of the school, whereby a certain sport is more popular and high profile in a given conference or area; or (3) a sport may be the revenue- generating one at the institution, and physician presence is preferred.

Care is a different component of service, and is expected to be provided equally to all student-athletes, regardless of gender, sport or any other criteria. Whatever you do, when negotiating to be a team physician for an organization that offers multiple sports for both genders, be sure to think equity! Do not ever offer a plan that neglects one gender or any single team. Offering to provide care for some and not others is not only unethical, it can be seen as being illegal under Title IX federal government standards, and likely will not even be entertained by the organization receiving your offer. Be prepared to provide services to all, and if you are unable to do so, then you must understand why an organization is not able to come to an agreement for your services. Ultimately, it is not about what you want to do or can do as a team physician; rather, it is about the services that the organization feels that they need to provide quality, accessible, and equitable care and coverage.

The high school sports level is similar to college with respect to prioritizing coverage, but is more focused on providing equal care to all. In reality, however, the majority of actual time commitment is with football game coverage. Between game coverage and physicals, one can spend between 150 to 200 hours over the course of a year.

When one examines the time and cost analysis of the Olympic sport coverage, the physician is often covering events nationally and internationally. This can become overwhelming in cost of time because of distances that must be traveled to foreign countries. There are often 1 or 2 week intervals, but they are non-revenue–generating, and typically only your travel and meal accommodations are cared for. The major advantages associated with the privilege of being selected to serve in such a capacity will be derived afterwards in the methods you choose to disseminate your involvement at that elite level to your potential patient clientele.

Through informal conversations, a professional football team physician stated that he is on the phone with the coach, athletic trainer, or general manager every day throughout the day during the season. This is also very common throughout high school, college, professional, and Olympic sports. It takes a lot of planning to be able to balance this commitment with the rest of your practice. The final cost of time that you must understand and evaluate is the fact that you will need to be available, if not in person, at least by phone, at all times for player-related issues. Coaches and administrators who need medical advice or assistance for things other than player's issues will call you because you become the medical point of contact for their organization. At some levels of sport this is, as they say, 24/7.

To offset some of the negative time-benefit factors, there are ways to minimize the time away from family and make this a positive experience, and not just for your professional endeavors. For example, you can include your family as often as possible with sporting events. Take your spouse and children to the games or events. Include them in the VIP aspects that are afforded to you by the team. If done right, that will make your time spent with a team a more inclusive experience for you and your family. Be sure that your family has such interest and that you are not "dragging them along."

This can also provide them with a better understanding of exactly what your role is, so that the times you are away from home with a team your family can appreciate your involvement.

It is impossible to quantify, but one of the real value added intangibles to being a team physician is the recognition and public perception of you because of your role.

Recognition in this manner, right or wrong, is the perception by the general public that you are the best because you were chosen to become the team physician. The "limelight" has improved many team physician's image in others' eyes, and the "ego factor" weighs heavily as a clear benefit. Your stature in the community, as perceived by the public and the media, is clearly enhanced, whether it is just locally at a high school, broadened with college or professional coverage, and even globally in some instances with professional and Olympic sports.

Not only is your stature enhanced with the public, but it is also enhanced among your colleagues, especially when you flash your team's logo to show that you are someone who is recognized as the chosen person by that team. As you stand or sit on the sidelines and become recognized by the fans of that organization as someone associated with the team, the benefit is clear. If by chance the event is televised and you are seen on national television and recognized in your role as team physician, people may perceive you as an elite physician. It is difficult to put a number on the value of these things, but ultimately it is a clear benefit financially.

While you bask in the limelight, don't forget the downside of this recognition. Dealing with elite or well-known athletes is a double-edged sword. Clearly, when your name is being associated with well-known athletes and you achieve good outcomes, then the result is a positive one. In the event that there is an untoward result, however, this could damage your reputation and your practice. A bad result or lawsuit that gets public attention can have far-reaching negative results financially and with job satisfaction, public perception, stress, and ego.

Your position of being a team physician, in virtually all instances, will enhance your practice by attracting more patients wanting to be treated by you, thereby increasing your business because you are perceived as an expert. This benefit is threefold: (1) often you will increase your overall volume of patients; (2) you may be able to narrow the scope of what you treat, which will allow you to focus on what you enjoy treating the most; and (3) patients are usually more inclined to accept what you tell them as being credible. Its hard to quantify the last, but don't underestimate the benefit of people's perception of you being on a higher level playing field than your competitors. Those pictures on the wall and the nice things prominent athletes and individuals say about you do not go unnoticed. Taking care of a team and being publicly recognized for that is some of the best and easiest marketing that exists. As they say in the MasterCard ads, it is "priceless."

Another direct financial benefit, regardless of the level of serving as a team physician, is the fee-for-service reimbursement recovered from the athletes who are seen and treated in your clinical setting or through surgical interventions. In professional sports, this is Workman's Compensation and almost always covered by insurance. In colleges, high schools, and Olympic sports, a significant number of athletes are uninsured or underinsured, creating a dilemma, because you may incur the liability and cost of doing business and receive no compensation for your services. This may be coupled with the problem of getting studies and procedures done at the institution where you work in what you, the sports team officials, the athlete, and possibly the parents, consider to be a timely manner. Often facility owners will not cooperate and will not agree to provide services at no charge simply because the patient is an athlete who you have a responsibility and contractual obligation to care for. Most times, simply waiting for preauthorization from an athlete's insurance provider to have an imaging study performed is in a timely manner is completely out of the question, leading to nonreimbursable services. This is frustrating because you feel you are providing optimal health care and making quality medical decisions in the best interest of the patient athlete. At the college level, some schools are willing to provide a portion of the reimbursement for uninsured or underinsured athletes. If the colleges have these arrangements, consider them helpful, because they can offset your incurred expenses elsewhere that are unaccounted for within the team physician–organization relationship. It is important to help create these arrangements where they do not exist. It is also a good idea to inquire about the details of what type of secondary athletic insurance plan a college might have for their student athletes.

At the high school level, there are a few programs that have been developed around the country to cover the uninsured athletes. These are not widespread because of the amount of time, energy, and sheer difficulty in developing an organization that can accomplish this goal. Although the end product is great, the commitment to make this happen is immense on the front end, and to sustain on an ongoing basis throughout the process.

Because you have seen the associated costs that go with the job, you must carefully evaluate all financial factors, even though there are huge financial benefits to being a team physician. Take a step back and ask yourself some basic, yet important questions:

Why is one person or group chosen to take care of a given team or organization?

How do you become that person?

How do you maintain that position if you are chosen?
What politics must I be aware of? Do I know the "real story"?
How much is money driving this decision?
Do I have others who I can trust to confide in for reviewing a contract?
Do I know who the decision-makers are?
Can I truly provide the services that are needed?

These are just some of many questions that need to be addressed before jumping into the role of a team physician. Remember, the people choosing you are doing so mostly on their perception of you, or perhaps because of mutual existing relationships. There are very few actual criteria to help them make their decision. The reality is that most of the decision-makers don't have enough hard knowledge to make a credible decision, mostly because a measuring stick does not exist. Interestingly, however, the system still works pretty well.

What is available to help people decide on a team physician? As an older physician, I will always recommend experience. My younger friends would use the old adage, "Hire old lawyers and young doctors." The American Orthopedic Society for Sports Medicine (AOSSM) published a pamphlet on this in 2005 called "Principles of Selecting Team Medical Coverage" [1]. The standard of quality guidelines are

1. The selection of a team physician should be based fundamentally on the physician's credentials and ability to provide the highest level of care available.
2. The process of selecting the team physician should include input from multiple parties that have an interest in the well-being of the players.
3. The selection of team medical staff should not be based on financial incentives offered by the physician and/or his or her institution.
4. The team should fully disclose any sponsorship, advertising or financial arrangement that the medical staff (or their institution) have made with the team.
5. The team and medical staff should ensure appropriate communication (within legal limitations) to players, other medical providers and management to provide for a more open understanding regarding the health care environment.

I have found two sources to be invaluable. One is a position letter by former Commissioner Tagliabue of the NFL (Paul Tagliabue, written communication, September 7, 2004) and the other is one by Commissioner Selig of Major League baseball (Allen H. Selig, written communication, November 17, 2004). Although these two elite organizations have taken the position of prohibiting sponsorship dollars from influencing the choosing of a team physician, this is not the norm, and unfortunately most professional teams are still letting marketing people drive their medical care decision-making process. In a lot of cases, this also has become the norm at the college and high school levels nowadays. What must be addressed is the ethical dilemma that exists when faced with these circumstances. It is in all of our best interest to work to try to get the NFL and Major League Baseball guidelines applied to all sports at all levels.

At this time in our competitive industry, more and more qualified sports medicine physicians are being trained, and these issues will likely continue to be hotly debated amongst us. This is a good thing, because it is important that we work together to devise appropriate and possibly even standardized guidelines to follow. If there are two equally qualified candidates for a team physician job, who gets appointed? Is it the person with the best connections and network? Is it the person with the best access to provide with marketing dollars? Is it the person who happened to know the owner, administrator, or worked with the athletic trainer on a previous occasion? Or is it the person with the strongest qualifications and ability to be most accessible?

This also raises the question of who is the most qualified and the manner in which this is determined. Our industry is continually being scrutinized and evaluated, but there are few credible mechanisms with which to compare physicians. The AOSSM has this high on its priorities, and will likely play a major role to help with developing guidelines for the decision-making. It is incumbent on all of us to understand and be engaged in this evolving process. If you take the position that you are not concerned about the money, then the very best way to minimize the financial aspects of being a team physician is to understand thoroughly all of the risks and benefits.

Once an analysis is completed, the real question we must all ask ourselves is, "Why did I go into sports medicine?" Although it is important to be able to assess and understand the financial issues, they should not be the driving force behind our decisions. If you make good, informed decisions, they will help you enjoy the practice of sports medicine and have a fulfilling career, regardless of the costs associated with being a team physician.

ETHICAL CONSIDERATIONS

The ethics of being a team physician are closely tied to the financial aspects, and must be considered as you evaluate the opportunities. Because the sum total of the financial rewards can be very high, careful attention to ethical behavior must be paid. Although the NFL and Major League Baseball have clear guidelines regarding the behavior of buying a sponsorship to become the team physician, nearly every other situation encountered in serving as a team physician has no guidelines or formal ethical standards to adhere to. The AOSSM has published "Principles for Selecting Team Medical Coverage" to assist individuals with such decisions [1]. This document serves as a good starting point for continued discussion to further expand upon the existing guidelines.

THE BOTTOM LINE

Up until this point we have primarily discussed the general considerations associated with fiscal operations of being a team physician. We have not yet identified any true, hard figures that define a monetary contractual relationship. The direct cost of your time being a team physician is easier to calculate if your obligations and the team's expectations are made clear from the outset.

As an active team physician at any level of sport, you must be able to realistically assess the time commitment necessary to do the job well and make sure you can commit to the obligation that you agree to.

As we expand our understanding of the financial aspects of being a team physician, it will be helpful to understand the entire landscape of actual salaries and fees paid by institutions, so that comparison and analysis can be done. This may be difficult to obtain because of the reluctance of the involved parties to share this information. To date, there is no vehicle to ascertain such information in a formal manner. Ultimate sharing of financial arrangements could in fact lead to a more positive working relationship between physicians and organizations, because unethical financial arrangements and behaviors would likely be minimized. As we expand our financial knowledge, we need to find a way to share the knowledge and experience of those who have established these programs and to disseminate this information. Although the direct financial benefits are relatively easy to quantify, the amount is extremely variable with different sports, because of the number and severity of injuries and the variations in compensation.

To clearly develop a value of worth for team physician services, the list in Box 1 should serve as a basis for items to consider.

Regarding direct financial benefits, the first and easiest one to evaluate is at the professional level. These arrangements are extremely variable and difficult to get information about. In some extreme circumstances, team physicians are paid by professional teams, have all of their expenses covered, and additionally receive additional support or stipend for malpractice coverage. From the information I have gathered, this is not the case across the board, and more often these jobs are performed gratis, with some minimal reimbursement support of expenses incurred while providing these services. Occasionally, in colleges, there are small fees for the team physician, but this is not the norm. There are a few large colleges that employ the nonorthopedic team physician as a member of the university faculty or staff, but this is not true in the majority of the situations.

So what is this magical dollar figure that should equate to equitable remuneration? As you can see from the many negotiable items, as well as all of the possibilities that need to be determined when establishing a contractual relationship, there may not be one figure that fits all circumstances. If you were to hear a rumor that Dr. X was receiving $20,000 to be the team physician of a local university, you would likely fall into the trap that most others do and make judgment on the basis of the dollar amount alone. Whether you believe the amount is too much or too little, you probably do not know any of the other components of the arrangement. This is the very reason why it remains so difficult to share contractual details with others in the profession. The bottom line is, no matter how much medical qualifications should be the foundation for serving as a team physician, the business aspects will ultimately secure relationships. As a result, revealing inner details of contractual negotiations are not in the best interest of either party.

Box 1: Basis for value of team physician services

- *Base salary*
- *Amount of time required as a team physician*
  Total number of athletes
  Game coverage requirements
  On-site clinic requirements
  Travel requirements
  Type of availability and accessibility
- *Time taken away from seeing billable patients in clinic*
- *Time taken away from operating*
- *Advertisement trade value*
- *Agreeable "official" or "exclusive" status*
- *Percent of athletes insured*
  Likelihood of receiving third-party reimbursement
  Secondary insurance coverage possibility
  Percent of Workman's Compensation
  Capitated services
  Percent of insured within approved regional network
- *Liability insurance coverage*
- *Methods of contractual evaluation, length of contract*
- *Responsibility for on-site supplies needed*
- *Supervision of athletic training staff by law*
- *Penalty and guidelines for termination of contract by either party*
- *Potential surgical cases*
- *Potential billing opportunities (ie, imaging, casting, and so on)*

In general, it is very satisfying to treat healthy, motivated athletes whose main goal is to get well and return to sport. These individuals are less likely to have accompanying complicated medical problems and the sequelae that go along with aging, poor health, and multiple diseases. This isn't to say that you won't come across such cases or don't need to be able to recognize them within the athletic population. In general, however, orthopedic decisions can be isolated to the injury at hand.

SUMMARY

Remember, time is the greatest negative financial burden that you accept as a sports medicine physician, because the only way to produce revenue as a physician is with your time. This time cost in doing business as a team physician can be high. Unless being a team physician is very rewarding to you through personal satisfaction or the other intangible indirect benefits associated with the role, being a team physician may not be a good financial decision for you as a person and a physician, or for your practice and your family.

Acknowledgments

I thank JK, MM, and the publishers for their willingness to help shed light and knowledge on these difficult subjects related to being a team physician. Also thanks to my many friends and colleagues for their insight on this subject.

Reference

[1] The American Orthopaedic Society for Sports Medicine (AOSSM). Principles for selecting team medical coverage. Rosemont, IL: AOSSM; 2005.

Clin Sports Med 26 (2007) 243–251

CLINICS IN SPORTS MEDICINE

SEVIER
UNDERS

Educational Opportunities and Implications Associated with the Team Physician

Robb S. Rehberg, PhD, ATC, CSCS, NREMT[a],*,
Joelle Stabile Rehberg, DO[b],
Michael Prybicien, MA, ATC, CSCS, NREMT[c]

[a]Department of Exercise and Movement Sciences, William Paterson University,
300 Pompton Road, Wightman Gymnasium, Wayne, NJ 07470, USA
[b]Montville Primary Care Physicians, 350 Main Road, Montville, NJ 07045, USA
[c]Passaic Board of Education, 101 Passaic Avenue, Passaic, NJ 07055, USA

O pportunities for physicians to teach others are not unique to sports medicine. Physicians in every medical discipline are involved in teaching at some level, whether it is in the classroom, at the bedside, in the office, or in the operating room. Of all the medical specialties, however, sports medicine may offer physicians the widest variety of educational opportunities. The sports medicine setting presents unique circumstances for physicians to be involved in education. Sports medicine physicians have the opportunity to teach a wide variety of individuals from diverse backgrounds and educational levels. This education takes on a variety of forms and covers a wide assortment of topics and experiences. This is a continual process that often begins with pre-participation physical examinations, continues with mechanism of injury and the treatment and rehabilitation process, and eventually ends with either a return to play, or in some circumstances, the disqualification from certain sport activities. Educating others is a challenging yet essential role of a team physician. This article examines the educational responsibilities of the team physician, educational opportunities in the sports environment, and methods and challenges to establishing a learning environment.

EDUCATIONAL OPPORTUNITIES OF THE TEAM PHYSICIAN

Teaching and the practice of medicine are inseparable. After all, team physicians should not forget that "doctor" is the Latin term for teacher. In the sports medicine setting, the audience can be anyone, and the lesson can also occur almost anywhere, and opportunities will present themselves in both formal and informal situations. The lesson may be in the traditional setting of the lecture

*Corresponding author. E-mail address: rehbergr@wpunj.edu (R.S. Rehberg).

0278-5919/07/$ – see front matter
doi:10.1016/j.csm.2007.01.004
© 2007 Elsevier Inc. All rights reserved.
sportsmed.theclinics.com

hall with a set topic and a defined audience. It can also occur in the office setting during a typical day of patient visits, at athlete pre-participation physical examinations, or an injury clinic conducted at a school. Educational opportunities often present themselves on the field of play while the game is in progress. In these situations, the audience may be anyone involved, whether it is the injured athlete, the inquisitive coach, the concerned parent, or the curious student. Thus, education of students (including athletic training, physical therapy, medical, and the like), residents, fellowship physicians, athletes, parents, administrators, coaches, and others is one of the core duties of the team physician [1].

Patient Education (Athletes)

Although every patient visit involves teaching to some degree, team physicians frequently find themselves in situations outside the average patient encounter. Beginning with the pre-participation examination, physicians have the opportunity to identify potential health risks and issues. This is an opportunity to educate athletes on important topics such as steroid use, eating disorders, proper flexibility and strengthening routines and concepts, menstrual irregularities, and obesity. Using the pre-participation as an educational session allows the team physician to provide important information to young adults who may otherwise not receive it. Ultimately, these lessons can serve as a valuable tool in the prevention of illness and injury.

In the sports medicine setting, patient education does not end with the office visit. The team physician can expect to be called on for advice in the athletic training room or on the sideline as well. Though this form of patient contact is usually informal and often brief, the value of these encounters shouldn't be underestimated; oftentimes athletes will approach the physician on the sideline with a question that may otherwise go unanswered.

Public Education

In addition to educating athletes, team physicians are responsible for educating other groups, such as coaches, parents, and school administrators. In many cases, the team physician is a highly visible member of the athletics staff, and is considered the authority on injury prevention and health and medical issues. For this reason, team physicians are often called upon to address coaching staffs and parent groups. This is a valuable opportunity for the team physician to educate the masses on injuries and illness in the athlete, dispel myths that can commonly cause confusion in the care of the athletic injuries, and introduce parents to the sports medicine team and its key members. In some instances these opportunities can also serve as an asset to the physician's practice in terms of advertisement and public relations.

Educating coaches on topics such as proper stretching, conditioning, and hydration can have a significant impact on an athletic program. As times have changed, the way the athlete is cared for has also changed. Some coaches, however, still follow the "old school" or "no pain, no gain" approach to coaching. It is crucial that coaches understand the current thinking regarding issues such as proper hydration, stretching, and weight loss. It is important to emphasize that the goal of sports medicine is not to influence coaching strategy or style, rather it is to enhance athlete performance through prevention of injuries and illnesses, immediate care, and safe return to play. Some coaches may also hesitate to refer athletes to the team physician for fear that the athlete may unnecessarily be withheld from participation. It is for this reason that team physicians establish an open line of communication with coaches, as well as educate them on the difference between the sports medicine approach and other conservative or more traditional approaches. Although challenging, it is important that all members of the sports medicine team, coaches included, are on the same page and have the athletes' best interests in mind.

In today's society, with the ever-growing industry of personal training, sport-specific training, and speed and agility schools, it has become even more necessary for sports medicine physicians to educate parents on training regimens and injury prevention. The true goal of a sports medicine professional is to prevent injuries to athletes. Physicians should educate parents on sport-specific topics as related to the age of the athlete through lectures, clinics, and direct contact. Some examples to keep in mind are plyometric training as related to age, and pitch counts as related to the little league baseball player.

Although the focus of medical education for the team physician is injury prevention and treatment, it is equally important to educate school administrators regarding the benefits of developing and implementing a sports medicine team. Physicians must educate administrators on the importance of certified athletic trainers, certified strength and conditioning specialists, nutritionists, sport psychologists, and various other sports medicine specialty physicians who will help decrease the rate of injuries of the athletes, improve athletic performance, and reduce the school's cost for medical liability insurance.

Clinical Education

One of the more obvious teaching situations in which team physicians participate involves clinical education of medical residents and students and students in allied health professions, including students in athletic training education programs, physical therapy, and nursing programs. Team physicians may have varying levels of involvement in formal educational programs, ranging from serving as a consultant or preceptor in the field, to clinical instructor or more formal academic appointments. Accredited athletic training education programs, for instance, require that a medical director be directly involved in the academic preparation of athletic training students. Team physicians who are associated with different professional education programs are faced with teaching students of varying educational levels and backgrounds. It is essential that physicians have a thorough understanding of each student's educational level and preparation. The challenge comes with understanding each student's level of education and meeting them at levels that provide a meaningful learning experience.

Although the importance of traditional classroom preparation is understood, many valuable educational opportunities occur outside of the classroom.

Valuable educational opportunities can occur in the medical office setting, although a busy practice can oftentimes hinder meaningful learning for students. Depending on the setting, some team physicians participate in weekly injury clinics conducted on location at schools they cover. Like the office setting, these situations can be valuable educational experiences for students, and allow more time for interaction between patient and student than in the office setting.

The operating room is another valuable educational venue for students. Direct surgical visualization of the anatomy of an injury, along with physician-led discussion, exposes students to anatomy and pathology in ways that cannot be matched by textbooks and classroom discussion. Moreover, cadaver dissection, in which students actively participate under supervision of a physician, enhances learning and builds upon knowledge gained in the classroom. During cadaver dissection laboratories, students, under the direct supervision of a physician, can be exposed to the anatomy in a manner that cannot be matched by a textbook or classroom lecture. The student is able to visualize structures that were once only available to them in a two dimensional photograph. During cadaver laboratories, students are also able to dissect structures, and then perform evaluative special tests on the cadaver to compare the differences of injured versus uninjured body structures.

Workshops and laboratory practice are two other useful educational methods used by team physicians. Workshops and laboratory sessions, which are often informal in nature, can range in topic and delivery from injury evaluation or treatment labs to mock injury scenarios. Students benefit from physician-supervised workshops focusing on specific clinical examination skills and knowledge, and often enjoy the informal and low-stress learning environment. Topics can be broad in scope, such as range of motion testing, strength testing, and special test practice, or can focus on a specific treatment technique for a certain injury.

Of all the educational experiences in sports medicine, clinical field experiences (ie, on the sideline, courtside, matside, and so forth) can be among the most valuable educational lessons in a student's education. It is an opportunity for students to make the connection between academic preparation and clinical practice. It is in these situations that team physicians have the opportunity to create a "teachable moment" on the sideline, because students are in the unique situation of being able to witness mechanism firsthand, followed by initial evaluation and treatment. Arguably, sports medicine is one of only a handful of medical disciplines that can capture this experience.

When covering athletic events, the sports medicine team may be presented with difficult medical situations. Preparation is the key to ensuring the athlete receives the best possible care, and preparation should always be included in the educational process. Students should know the importance of emergency action plans and how they are implemented when they are covering athletic events. Mock scenarios and drills serve a dual purpose in that they educate students as well as prepare them to act in an emergency. Some examples are spine boarding of the injured athlete, dealing with acute heat illness, and lightning storm safety (controlling game action), to name a few.

Naturally, the topics team physicians usually teach are related to the practice of sports medicine; however, lessons often reach far beyond injuries and illnesses. Although the focus of the students' education is on medical knowledge and skills, there is an ever-growing importance for the team physician to focus on medical ethics and decision-making, health care administration and billing, and regulatory affairs. These topics are all essential to the professional preparation of students pursuing careers in sports medicine. Team physicians should be aware of these, and be prepared to discuss and answer questions on these subjects. This is especially true for physicians who serve as mentors for medical students, residents, and fellowship physicians. The goal of the attending physician is to provide an educational experience that will best prepare his student to practice medicine independently.

Physicians may use a variety of ways to help students understand the issues dealing with medical ethics and decision-making. Of course, leading by example is quite possibly the best method. Actively involving students in the medical review process, in which the student assists the physician in reviewing a case for a medical insurance company, attorney, or workers' compensation case manager, allows the student to review another physician's decision- making process and form his own opinions as to whether the physician's actions were medically ethical.

In the ever-changing world of medical insurance, it is more important than ever that medical students understand that medicine is a just as much a business as it is a science. Students from all disciplines must gain experience in dealing with medical coding (ICD-9 and CPT), insurance pre-certification and authorization, and proper medical documentation. Physicians should use their support staff in educating students about each of these topics, and allow them to spend time with the office managers and other key staff members to gain a better understanding of the daily operation of the practice.

Physicians who are fortunate enough to be involved with sports medicine fellowships find themselves in a wonderful opportunity to serve as mentors to younger physicians interested in establishing increased skill, expertise, and networking in the field of sports medicine. It is important for fellowship directors to recognize that teaching clinical skills is not the only benefit of a fellowship. Furthermore, assigning a fellowship physician to a school or team and simply assuming that he or she will just fit right in is a big mistake. The "MD" or "DO" after one's name does not automatically mean competency in sports medicine, and assuming so is a recipe for failure. Granted, the fellowship is an opportunity for learning to occur; however, to the athletes and the medical staff affiliated with the program, it is serious business. Everyone, including the fellowship physician, must be prepared and understand how to fit into a role beyond simply showing up. Exposing a fellow to the environment, the people, and the protocols associated with the program ahead of time will prove rewarding and beneficial to everyone involved.

Research and Professional Education

Aside from the traditional educational opportunities available to students in the sports medicine setting, participation in research can be a valuable and rewarding educational activity. Of course, educating other members of the medical community and contributing to the body of medical knowledge through publishing and presenting original research is the primary reason for conducting research; however, physicians should also encourage students to develop a curiosity for research and promote involvement in research activities whenever possible. Including students in scientific research, clinical trials, case studies, and presentations at professional conferences aids in bolstering the student's knowledge of the subject matter as well as introducing the student to the world of research. In some cases, a student's involvement in research activity may instill a penchant for research that may turn today's student into tomorrow's scientist.

CHALLENGES TO ESTABLISHING A LEARNING ENVIRONMENT IN THE SPORTS MEDICINE SETTING

Education is an essential part of being a team physician, but it's not always easy. Several challenges to teaching in the sports medicine setting often arise; however, many of these challenges are easily overcome with experience. The effective team physician is one who anticipates these challenges and prepares accordingly.

Although hands-on clinical education is a valuable part of a student's educational experience, some patients may be uncomfortable with student involvement in their care. Although many patients welcome the attention, some may interpret student involvement as receiving substandard care, or as an invasion of privacy. Others may become impatient with the extended amount of time it takes for an evaluation to be completed. Still others may be uneasy or unwilling to allow a student to perform a certain test or procedure (particularly if a gender difference exists), even in the presence of the physician. Team physicians should always communicate clearly with their patients regarding student involvement, in order to defuse any apprehension regarding the patient-doctor-student encounter. Conversely, team physicians must also stress that the student maintain strict confidentiality regarding each patient encounter.

In some cases, the situation may not allow an adequate opportunity for student involvement in a patient's care. This often occurs during game situations in which assessment, diagnosis, and return-to-play decisions must be completed quickly. The team physician must balance the educational needs of the student with the needs of the athlete in a game situation. Likewise, the fast pace of a busy medical office may not always allow for meaningful learning for a student. Often a physician's full schedule in the office may not allow time for direct student involvement or discussion in every case. In these situations, the physician should emphasize that learning can occur by careful observation of physician-patient interaction. As with experiences on the field, physicians must find a way to balance the needs of the student with the demands of a busy practice.

Adapting to different learning styles can be challenging for any teacher. Some students will be auditory learners and benefit from lecture and discussion. Other students may be visual learners and learn by example through demonstration in the clinical setting. Still others may be kinesthetic learners and learn by doing. The challenge for any clinical instructor is to recognize different learning styles and present material in a way that best meets the needs of the student. This can be especially difficult when teaching several students at once. By balancing lecture, demonstration, and practice, the physician can address the needs of all learners.

Too often, students tend to compartmentalize knowledge learned in the classroom, and fail to make the link between what they have learned about anatomy, physiology, and pathology, and what they are presented with in the field. This compartmentalization of knowledge can be a barrier a student's true understanding of the injury or illness process. Learning over time, a concept now used in athletic training education, helps combat compartmentalization of knowledge by introducing and reintroducing topics in increasingly greater depth throughout the educational process. Team physicians should embrace the learning-over-time concept, and challenge students to make the connection between what they have learned in each of their classes to the cases they are presented with in the field.

FACILITATING LEARNING IN THE SPORTS MEDICINE SETTING

Teaching may be second nature to some physicians. Others may be uncomfortable with their roles as teachers. Regardless of comfort level, physicians can increase their effectiveness as teachers by first considering how best to facilitate a learning environment in their particular practice. Although every practice setting is different, the following are points that team physicians should consider that can help facilitate learning in the sports medicine setting.

Lead by Example

Team physicians routinely work outside the office setting and are thus highly visible to the public. While working on the sidelines, teaching and leading by example take on new meaning as the team physician practices before dozens and sometimes thousands of spectators. Factors such as professional dress, demeanor, and punctuality are essential in teaching by example and for setting the tone for the educational environment in the field. Team physicians should also strive to make themselves approachable, and actively engage in conversation with students, the sports medicine staff, coaches, and others.

Understanding your Audience

All students and all professional education programs are not created equal. It is imperative that team physicians have an understanding of their students' educational discipline as well as their level of education. Each student may have a different understanding of the topic being discussed. For example, the medical resident should have a firm knowledge of the medications used in the athlete who has hypertension; whereas the athletic training student may be aware of the medications, but not be familiar with how they are to be used. Being able to share information with students without discouraging them is an essential aspect of teaching as the team physician.

Recognize the Value of a Multidisciplinary Approach

The teaching team physician must take a multidisciplinary approach to teaching. Although the majority of sports medicine topics are orthopedic in nature, some of the more important sports medicine pearls involve general medicine. A strong general medical background is essential for the teaching team physician, and the importance of thorough general medical evaluation skills should never be underestimated. An understanding of general medical conditions such as the athlete who has asthma, diabetes, hypertension, and how to evaluate for them is just as important as evaluating an orthopedic condition. Knowledge in other specialty areas such as internal medicine, neurology, cardiology, dermatology, and pediatrics as they relate to sports medicine is also essential to the team physician in the role of teacher.

Encourage Dialog Among Members of the Sports Medicine Team

Learning is a two-way street. Although the team physician is usually the teacher, each member of the sports medicine team possesses his own unique perspective, experience, and expertise. The information that can be shared by individuals such as athletic trainers, strength and conditioning specialists, physical therapists, nurses, resident physicians, and students should be appreciated, because their viewpoints can provide a refreshing outlook. Each member of the sports medicine team must know his or her limitations and realize the importance of the sports medicine team approach. Likewise, each member of the sports medicine team should be willing to share knowledge as well as learn from others. A sports medicine team that is comprised of health and medical professionals willing to work together, share, and learn from each other allows for the best possible care of the athletes they serve.

Be Prepared

The team physician should always be ready for a learning experience, because a teaching opportunity can occur anywhere and at anytime. When students are present, the physician must view the patient encounter as more than just a clinical procedure. In many situations, the physician can transform even the most routine evaluation or procedure into a teachable moment. The effective teaching team physician is able to recognize these opportunities, which routinely occur in the office and on the field.

The team physician should also look to take advantage of "down time" and create teaching moments. While covering an athletic event, such down time can occur during pre-game activities, half-time, time-outs, and while traveling to and from the event. These are all examples of opportunities for meaningful educational discussion between the team physician, sports medicine staff, and students.

There may be times where the team physician may not have all the answers. Often a physician's first instinct may be to work through the topic without admitting he or she does not know the answer; however, admitting unfamiliarity with a topic and following up after further research lends credibility to the physician as a teacher. As in any other medical discipline, there is a wealth of knowledge available through textbooks, journals, and online sources. The team physician should use these resources to his or her advantage when serving as a teacher.

SUMMARY

Teaching is one of the primary responsibilities of the team physician. After all, teaching and medicine are inseparable. Educating others is a challenging yet essential role of a team physician, and understanding the educational opportunities, responsibilities, and methods of creating a learning environment are essential qualities of the team physician. The successful teaching team physician is the one who accepts the role of an educator, understands the importance of involvement in the educational process at all levels, and is able to create an environment conducive to student learning, while at the same time serving as a valuable resource for patients, coaches, administrators, and the public.

Reference

[1] Team physician consensus statement. Am J Sports Med 2000;28:440–2.

Clin Sports Med 26 (2007) 253–263

CLINICS IN SPORTS MEDICINE

SEVIER
UNDERS

Marketing Ideas and Strategies for Building Upon the Team Physician's Role

Jim Clover, MEd, ATC, PTA*, Jerome Wall, MD

The S.P.O.R.T. Clinic, 4444 Magnolia Avenue, Riverside, CA 92501, USA

"**S**how me the money" is without question the number one reason to market and advertise. That may sound silly to say, but look at some of the advertising and it will then be time to question and understand the thought process of those that advertise and market. In this article, the authors attempt to provide information on marketing and advertising that will help your business, and that we hope will provide some thought-provoking ideas for you to pursue that will enable you to increase your company's bottom line and "show them the money."

The average American is inundated with over 3700 advertising messages per day. The key to successful marketing is to make your advertisement the one that counts—the one everyone will remember when they need the service or product you provide.

The best marketing and advertising takes advantage of all of the senses, not just what we read or see. Next time you go to Disneyland check out how they are able to use sound, (background music), smell (food), touch, sight, color, and interaction (using your brain) to sell their products; they are very good. The patients/clients are using their senses in your office; you can either be the person in charge of them or ignore them. Remember that ignoring them or not doing anything is a decision.

ALWAYS REMEMBER YOUR MARKET AND ADVERTISE TO INCREASE REVENUE

Names

What's in a name? Short names like Nike, Coke, Sears, Target, and so forth make a lot more sense, because the consumer can remember them and that is what it is all about. Longer names can sometimes be shortened with an acronym. For example, "Sport Physiology Orthopedic Rehabilitation and Treatment" can simply be referred to as S.P.O.R.T. Rhyming and alliteration can

*Corresponding author. E-mail address: sportclinic@earthlink.net (J. Clover).

0278-5919/07/$ – see front matter
doi:10.1016/j.csm.2007.01.006

© 2007 Elsevier Inc. All rights reserved.
sportsmed.theclinics.com

also be effective, but keep in mind that the name should fit both the product and the style of the company (Fig. 1).

Brochures and Flyers

Go to a physician's office and look for the flyers and brochures. There may be an expensive glossy flyer with all the physicians' names, pictures, and backgrounds, or just business cards (Fig. 2). What happens to these expensive shiny brochures once the patients have them? Does anyone take one home? If so, what would he do with it—put it on the refrigerator and take down some more important child's artwork? Doubt it. This is trash right out the door. First, look at it. The pictures of the doctors look like none of them wanted to have their picture taken. Now what does this say to the consumer? How much did this cost to produce? Was the investment ever assessed in terms of its return? I think you know the answers to these questions.

Read the background information—does it answer the questions the consumers have, or is it what the physician wanted to say. Now this information it is very important, but what would be a better way to get this information to the public, so they could see it and if they wanted, could take it home and keep it for later use? How about some pictures on the wall, kind of a hall of fame of the group's physicians, doing things they enjoy at their work. Near the pictures, display information the patients might want to know, such as where the physician went to school, their success rate in surgery (outcomes), how they are continuing their education in the medical field, or papers or books they have published. Maybe even a visionary statement of where they see medicine going and how they are going to be a part of that vision. There would be a business card next to their picture that the consumer could take home, with a Web site where this information or an expanded version would be available. You could even have a baseball card for the physician, athletic trainer, or physical therapist, kind of corny maybe, but the consumer may keep it and show it around (Fig. 3). For those who don't have access to a computer, a kiosk setup with the

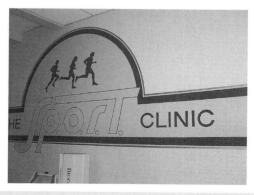

Fig. 1. Let there be no doubt who you are.

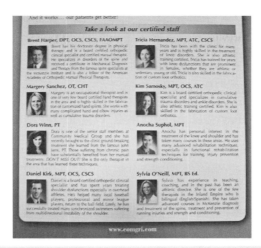

Fig. 2. High cost glossy brochure. (*Courtesy of* Jerome Wall, MD, Riverside, CA.)

company's name and Web site is a good alternative. This would be cheaper and better.

One of the authors of this article (JC) opened a store once, researched products, got prices, visited other stores, and then came up with a product line of

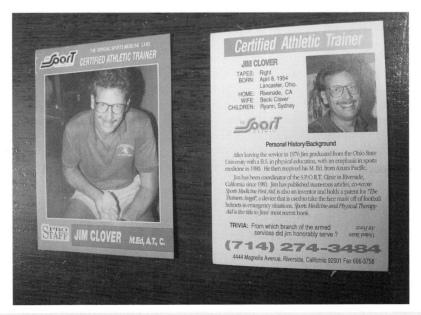

Fig. 3. Baseball card.

things that he just loved. What was wrong with this? It wasn't what the consumer wanted. Remember that.

So what is the difference between advertising and marketing? Advertising is the printed material, television, and radio commercial, whereas marketing is working with and through people.

CONSIDERATIONS WHEN SELLING YOUR PRODUCT
Advertising
Advertising is the activity of attracting public attention to a product or business, as by paid announcements in the print, broadcast, or electronic media.

Marketing
Many people believe that marketing is just about advertising or sales; however, marketing is everything a company does to acquire customers and maintain a relationship with them. Even the small tasks such as writing thank-you letters, playing golf with a prospective client, returning calls promptly, or meeting with a past client for coffee can be thought of as marketing. The ultimate goal of marketing is to match a company's products and services to the people who need and want them, and thereby ensure profitability. Being a team physician lends itself to many opportunities for indirect and direct marketing.

Logo
A logo is a great way for the public to recognize your company, one of the best out there may be Nike's. The logo can be a word in a certain kind of font or an art design. Some logos keep a standard color, whereas other may vary like a chameleon's with what their background. No matter what the color, stick to one logo. Multiple logos can become confusing to the customers. Take advantage of being on the sidelines and court if you are contractually working with a sports team or program by having identifiable clothing.

The phrase "Just do it" is automatically associated with Nike. Because it is so well-known, it is obvious that it has become a very successful slogan. Something like, "The Inland Empire's Answer to Your Sports Medicine Needs," may be a little long. The thing to remember is that the slogan should be all-inclusive of your product, while not holding it back from possible future growth or addition of other products.

Color
Color is important—look what Coke has done with red, or go to a major university and see what they can do. Go to a Michigan versus Ohio State football game and there will be no question whose side you are on by the colors worn. When determining a color scheme for a clinic, you need to consider what the color may mean to others. Make sure you don't take sides by the colors you have chosen, by picking one school's colors over another's. As funny as it seems, it may be a factor in a potential client's decision when buying the product or choosing your service (Fig. 4).

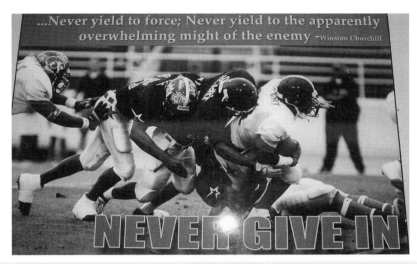

Fig. 4. All-Star Football Classic with logos on the jerseys. (*Courtesy of* Jim Clover, MEd, ATC, PTA, Riverside, CA.)

Billboard

Billboard advertisements can be static, like the ones that you see along the side of the road, or moving, like the name of your clinic on the side of a van (Fig. 5). You can also place it on a tent at large events (Fig. 6). Repeated name

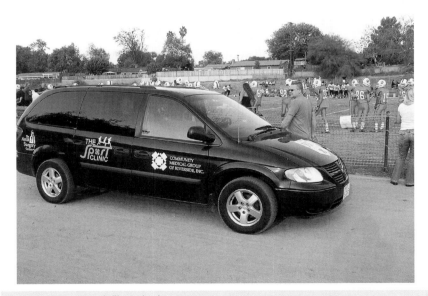

Fig. 5. Clinic name billboard advertising on a van at a sporting event.

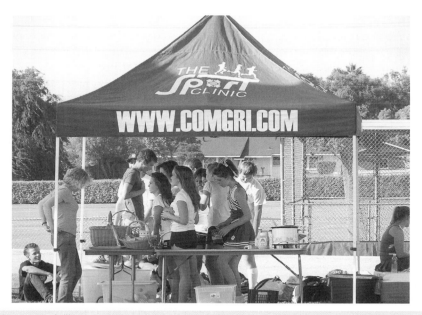

Fig. 6. Tent billboard advertising at an event, with Web domain name for extended marketing.

recognition is important, but its worth is hard to determine. Make your logo into a flag; the public cannot see your name enough—just look at what Nike or Gatorade has done; their names are everywhere.

Yellow Page Advertisement

You have to put something in the yellow pages or your target customers will never find you. Make something bold that draws positive attention to you. Outlining your advertisement will draw the consumer's eyes directly toward what you have to say. Make sure to include your Web site so the consumer has the ability to access more information. In most cases, a consumer will not make a sole judgment on a medical decision on what is said in the yellow pages, but placing an advertisement in the best yellow page book makes the customers want to try you.

Word of Mouth

Okay, word of mouth—is that marketing or advertising? Maybe a little of both. Everyone advertises that he is the best, with top-notch facilities, and great patient care. But actions speak louder than words. If a patient goes to your office and waits for hours in a waiting room, with old magazines, dirty chairs, close to sick people, and during his waiting time no one communicates with him about the reason for the wait, he will become frustrated and not value your services. Some customer may be impressed with the wait time, whereas others will look elsewhere very quickly and tell others, that tell others, that tell others, and you know how that goes. So, if you are advertising good service, you need to deliver. Everyone's time is equally valuable.

Web Site

A Web site is important in obtaining new customers. These sites vary tremendously with respect to how they look and what they do. Most medical establishments use them as promotional sites, and therefore when the site is established and upgraded, make sure to remember the main goal—to bring in patients and "show me the money." To ensure that the Web site will become an integrated part of your marketing, make sure to put it in front of the best prospects at the right times.

The Web site domain name is important. If you don't think so, just look at what some people are paying to get the one they want. Once again, the domain name is for your customer to remember, not necessarily the first letter of all the words in your name. The domain name, like everything else, should drive business to you. There are really no accidents in the consumer coming to your site.

When establishing a domain name for your Web site, don't force consumers to remember anything they don't have to; it just doesn't make sense. The name should be something related to your company that is easy to remember. Don't make the consumers work any harder than they have to remember how to get to you. Make sure that your logo is on the site, and that colors match your business colors.

Create a place on your Web site where customers can register to get more information, send you an e-mail, or receive an e-mail about updates or pertinent information for them specifically. Web sites have the ability to track where the interest is coming from. They can record the number of "hits" received, where they are coming from, and what pages are viewed the most.

The number of hits is not as important or useful as the pages viewed and the length of stay on those pages. It is more important to track the "session" than hits. A session is a unique visit by a single individual, whether she looks at one page or several pages. It is important to create a site that people will stay on for a long period of time. Make the site interactive, exciting, personal, and fun. Pictures are a great option because 85% of people are visually oriented.

What kind of Web site do you have? On interactive Web sites, the patient/consumers are able to download useful information, such as a rehabilitation protocol, or even register as patients online. Make sure your site is easy for visitors to navigate.

It is somewhat important to keep your site fresh with new information, but it is more important to keep the provided information pertinent and useful for your client/patient. Items to include on a Web site include the following:

- Information about the medical staff
    A resume or curriculum vita that can be downloaded by the patient
    Easy-to-read information about the physician, physical therapist, athletic trainer, and other staff members
- Any and all forms that can be downloaded and filled out before the appointment. This will save everyone time.
- Any educational information you may want for the patient or clients
    Your original work

A list of other Web sites they can visit for information—make sure they are not sites that will take business away from you. If you include sites about your physicians, check to make sure all the information is accurate, including proper credentials and addresses.

TRACKING YOUR MARKETING AND ADVERTISING

What brought you the money? If you cannot document and follow your advertising, you will be unable to support the significance of marketing and advertising. This is a responsibility of each individual to follow, not something to put off. Some examples follow:

The phone operator should randomly check and put in writing how a client got the number to call. Make sure this is random. For instance, the operator could ask two people in the morning and two in the afternoon. This doesn't sound like much, but in 1 week the operator will have asked 20 people and in a year, 1040 people. This is a real statistical number that can be factored into a marketing and advertising budget the next year.

When patients fill out the paperwork to get registered to see the medical practitioner, ask for referral sources. They can be categorized for statistical and analysis purposes. Categories can include the primary referral (friend, relative, commercial, newspaper ad, and so forth), and secondary referral (the name of the referral source).

Without following this information you will never find out what is working. This information will tell you where it is best to place your advertising dollars and show you where the money is coming from. This is imperative to do!

"Show me the money" can be achieved through the use of soft marketing that drives client/patients to you. These are thing like getting quoted in the local newspaper, school newspaper, magazine, and other publications, and network or cable television shows. Once again, it is very, very important to track and keep record of this. If there is a good article, put it in a frame or plaque format and mount it to the wall. This will add length to the marketing piece (Fig. 7).

Bring potential clients into your clinic through educational seminars, first aid, and cardiopulmonary resuscitation (CPR) classes, and allow groups to meet there. Be a positive part of your community. Establish and run an All-Star athletic event. Remember people only remember the last good thing you did, but they will remember a bad experience for a lifetime.

TRACKING AND MEASURING YOUR MEDIA COVERAGE

Media coverage adds value. Although many take this as a given, it's not always fully appreciated. The reason: it doesn't translate well to the bottom line. Questions such as where the news is published, how many people read it, and most important, the way in which messages are perceived all have a tangible impact on whether or not patients use your service or buy your product. But without a method for accurately collecting and analyzing such data, it's difficult to

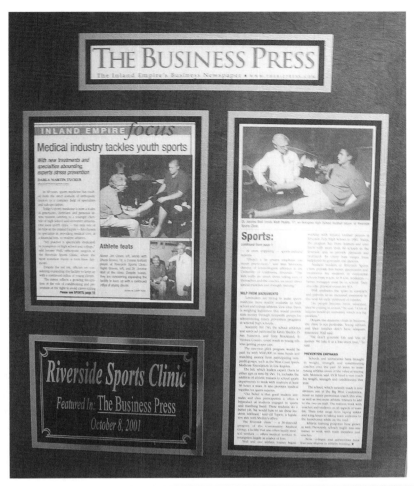

Fig. 7. Newspaper articles. (*Courtesy of* Press Enterprise Co., Riverside, CA; with permission.)

measure the effectiveness and impact of your efforts. Yet there are ways to measure this value—and not all of them are expensive or elaborate.

Do-it-Yourself Media Monitoring

Counting clips—the physical number of articles a company's name appears in—is the simplest measure for quantifying the success or failure of what you are doing. Knowing the number of stories (or hits) your company generates and how those numbers stack up against the competition offers a window into the recognition that a company has among reporters and those who follow the news.

Measuring and Analyzing Your Success

In addition to monitoring various media for clips, you'll also want to analyze your success. Measuring the true value of media coverage is a topic that continues to confound marketing and public relations (PR) executives throughout the world. The reason is simple: the task requires you to objectively analyze something that's largely subjective—a balanced article to one person may be a hatchet-job to another.

One traditional and largely objective method for measuring the value of an article is to assign it a monetary figure. This is done using "advertising value equivalency" (AVE). AVE assesses the value of an article by weighing it against the cost of related advertising space. The dollar figure is based on the publication's rate card. For example, a large, front-page advertisement is generally more expensive than a small, mid-publication ad.

Although AVE will give you some indication of the value of your exposure, it fails to recognize how the news was actually reported: Was the company portrayed in a favorable light?; What was the overall tone of the article?; What messages were picked up?; What's the enduring positive or negative effect on the brand?

Fortunately, as with media monitoring, there are computerized systems that automate much of the process, and in doing so, bring a measure of objectivity to the subjective data. These systems combine the features of an electronic clipping service with a series of algorithm-based measurements to capture, categorize, and assess company-specific coverage, as well as coverage of competitors and the industry at large. Media measuring systems offer three advantages:

1. Because each article is weighed according to a set of mathematical equations, the results are completely objective. Human frailties such as pride, insecurity, and anger are removed from the equation.
2. The predetermined set of measurements makes it very easy to compare coverage from different periods of time, PR campaigns, and messaging exercises, as well as between your company and its competition. The better-equipped media monitoring systems also provide the ability to drill down to specific criteria and determine whether one factor, such as publication type, has an impact on another, such as tonality of coverage. This depth of information can be extremely helpful in instances such as crisis situations, when companies may prefer to work with those reporters who generally issue more favorable coverage.
3. Automated measurement systems generate easy-to-understand, graphically enhanced reports that can be appreciated by those who don't have a PR background. Report information is condensed into color-coded bar graphs and pie charts that offer a simple yet effective representation of how your PR efforts contribute to your company's success.

Of course, there are some drawbacks to computerized measurement. The first is cost. Fortunately, with advances in technology, the price of automated measurement and analysis has dropped significantly, making it a viable option for more small businesses.

There's also an issue with the limitations of objectivity. Although the objectivity of automated measurement is one of its fundamental benefits, PR is still more art than science. So no matter how accurate the scoring system, the ultimate measure of PR is how the individual reader perceives the coverage.

There's little question that strategic, proactive PR can have a positive impact on a company's bottom line. For small businesses, the ability for PR to accelerate overall growth is even more substantial; however, if PR is done haphazardly with little regard for outcome (beyond scoring a hit), then much of the effort will be ineffective.

To get the most out of all your PR efforts, you should carefully consider the benefits of media monitoring and measurement and choose the system that best suits your company's immediate and long-range needs.

The bottom-line is that the advertising, marketing, and PR methods that you use need to be measured, because someday you will have to explain their effectiveness and importance, and "show them the money."

Clin Sports Med 26 (2007) 265–283

CLINICS IN SPORTS MEDICINE

SEVIER
UNDERS

Lessons in Sports Medicine: Advice from Experience

Edward G. McFarland, MD*, Peter A. Dobrowolski, BS,
Umasuthan Srikumaran, MD, Youxin Su, MD

Divisions of Sports Medicine and Shoulder Surgery, Department of Orthopaedic Surgery,
The Johns Hopkins University, 600 North Wolfe Street, Baltimore, MD 21287, USA

The best advice about sports medicine interventions comes from those who have been in the trenches—from those who have made some mistakes, as well as those who have had successful outcomes. To obtain such advice, we asked sports medicine physicians experienced in the management of sports teams to share their thoughts and ideas as a guide for residency- or fellowship-trained physicians entering the specialty. Although we acknowledge that other groups of sports-involved individuals, such as athletic trainers, could supply valuable information, we limited our requests to physicians so that we would have a manageable scope and specific focus for this report.

We sent e-mails to the members of the American Orthopaedic Society for Sports Medicine in the fall of 2006. Of the 1724 requests e-mailed, we received 92 (5.3%) responses. Those 92 respondents took care of major professional teams (28, 30.4%), minor league professional teams (32, 34.8%), collegiate teams (62, 67.4%), and secondary school or other athletic teams (60, 65.2%).

The advice given in the following pages should be read with the following caveats in mind. First, the information was not studied in a scientific manner, and the comments were edited only minimally. Second, we offered the contributors the right of anonymity to promote genuine responses and did not attempt to contact any contributor. We believe that the comments provided represent the writer's reality. Third, we did not perform any statistical analysis, so the information presented is level-5 information. Fourth, some of the advice offered is duplicated in other parts of this issue; such repetition should emphasize the importance of the given lessons, admonitions, or warnings. Lastly, these commentaries are purely subjective and are not intended in any way to constitute a standard of care or a legal standard. The guidance offered (divided into

*Corresponding author. Edward G. McFarland, MD, c/o Elaine P. Henze, BJ, ELS, Department of Orthopaedic Surgery, Johns Hopkins Bayview Medical Center, 4940 Eastern Avenue, #A672, Baltimore, MD 21224. *E-mail address:* ehenze1@jhmi.edu

0278-5919/07/$ – see front matter
doi:10.1016/j.csm.2007.01.007 © 2007 Elsevier Inc. All rights reserved.
sportsmed.theclinics.com

categories based on content) should be recognized as advice only and should not be taken as representations of scientific or legal standards.

ESTABLISHING A PRACTICE

First, you and your family should assemble several bullet points of the utopian practice and place to live. Consider family, lifestyle, and potential practice opportunities. Compare all of the opportunities and check off the bullet points. This method is an objective way of making a decision. Second, once you have moved to your area, set some defined practice goals and a plan on how you want to attain them. As long as they are morally and ethically sound, stay the course to reach your goals.

–John D. Campbell, MD

Taking care of a high school athletic program includes taking care of the entire community. Developing relationships at these athletic events is the best marketing tool available for your practice. It is better than covering a college or professional team because the community is a static reservoir of patients, not a transient flow.

–Jeff Traub, MD

Try to be involved with a team with which you might otherwise have a connection. For example, I have found it very rewarding to be a team physician for the local high school that my now-elementary-school-age kids will attend. This participation not only satisfies my desire to be involved as a team doc, but also creates a connection to my community that goes beyond the playing field. Remember, you won't fill your operating room schedule with athletes. However, their parents, grandparents, and friends will come to see you as patients and keep your schedule busy. Always be willing to talk to the coaches and the parents, buy ads in the school program, speak at career day, etc., to ingrain yourself in the community.

–Dan Gurley, MD

Beware of taking a job in a city solely for the purpose of taking care of a collegiate or professional athletic team or program. There are two reasons: first, the ownership or leadership of the team may change and you could be excused of your responsibilities, even if you have been doing the best job on the planet; second, your entire life will not be taking care of the team, and where you live and practice should be a place that you and your family want to live. If you or your family dislikes a location, you will, in the final analysis, have a good chance of being unhappy.

–Anonymous

Taking care of a team should be something that is performed out of love for sport. If one takes care of a team because he or she feels that it will give credibility or acclaim, it is for the wrong reason.

This job is truly a community service and should be viewed as such; otherwise, the decision-making process becomes entangled more in the win/loss aspect than in the general best interests of the patient. The pressures can be enormous, and if you cannot make the proper call because of outside pressures and you return an athlete to play too early, then the system has failed the patient at the most important time.

I have found the coverage issues to be both rewarding and frustrating. The rewards of seeing a player you have treated going on to a professional career or receiving a Division I scholarship are especially rewarding; however, the politics of a Division I school can take all the fun and excitement out of the coverage. I would recommend that each person who is thinking of providing coverage examine closely his or her motives and, if appropriate, try it. One will never regret the attempt.

–Joshua Siegel, MD

I have seen this scenario several times; it has not happened to me personally, but I have witnessed it. A young, newly trained, sports medicine surgeon arrives in town, and rather than build his practice and be patient in letting his skill and experience develop, he tries to "take over" and wrestle the teams from established surgeons who have been caring for said teams for years. This is a hole from which the young surgeon can never get out. Remember, as a physician new to a community or athletic program: always take the high road, and the cream does eventually rise to the top.

–Anonymous

Do not move to a university town and expect the physicians already taking care of the teams promised to you to leave without a fight. Any change in who is caring for the teams has to be agreed on at every level of the university–from the president, to the board of trustees, to the deans, to the athletic director, to the coach, to the head athletic trainer. Similarly, do not initiate a change in the team coverage unless you are ready to take some serious political heat. Physicians who have taken care of teams know board of trustee members who can exert significant pressure on the university through direct political means or by threatening to withdraw donations to the university or athletic program. My advice is to let the university come to you only after the political dirty dealing has been done or to find other compromises that might make all parties happy, or at least appeased.

–Anonymous

In initial discussions with the team, represent yourself as an objective physician. Do not get involved in any "opportunity" in which the ethics of the practice of medicine are compromised. Talk through different clinical scenarios, including return-to-play decisions, before they actually occur. You do not want your team relationship tied to making decisions that are not in a player's best medical interest.

–Dante Brittis, MD

In dealing with elite-level teams, it is important to keep in mind the fickle nature of the physician's relationship with the team. Things can change ever so quickly. If you base your identity on this relationship, you are risking a big fall. Do a good job, remain humble, and understand there is more in life. Also, go out of your way to keep the general manager and coaches informed personally. Don't rely on the athletic trainer to be the go-between.

—Anonymous

My mentors passed along simple advice that has worked well in several practice locations across the country: "Invest in yourself and your community, and success will follow" and "to understand the needs of the athlete, you must interact with them in their environment as well as yours." Take the time to be with your teams, athletes, and athletic trainers—not just during competitions but in the practice environment. Finally, be available; in their mind, the athlete has an emergency, so we must evaluate the problem as such.

—Paul R. Reiman, MD

I have been successful in building a practice taking care of high school athletes. Their parents closely observe how you take care of their child, and if you do a good job, you may quickly have 4 or 5 patients with the same last name. You won't find that at any other level.

—Frank Thomas, MD

Professional indoor soccer was a novel sport when I became team physician for the local franchise in 1984. It wasn't the glamour sport like the major pro sports. Because of the relative minor league nature of the sport, the players, coaches, and front office were low key and down to earth, with few big egos and a moderate salary structure. The time spent with the players and organization was time well spent. Because of the low pay, the players all coached multiple soccer teams as their primary source of income, with thousands of youth and select athletes under their control. Even though the pro franchise is now defunct, connections with the former players, coaches, and league officials provide a steady source of referrals to my practice. Moral to this story: national TV exposure is overrated and does not necessarily equate to long-term practice enhancement.

—Howard A. Moore, MD

PRIORITIES AND ETHICS

View the athletes as patients first and athletes second. Never let the athlete feel that you are altering their medical care to meet a spoken or unspoken team goal.

—Jo Hannafin, MD

Always keep the safety of the athlete as the number one priority, not the win/loss record of the team. Doing so may put you at odds with the coaching staff or front office, but in the end, they will respect you for it. You out rank the head coach on medical matters and have the sole responsibility of determining whether an athlete can play or not—do not take this responsibility lightly.

–Brian Crites, MD

Do not compromise your treatment because your patient is an athlete. Stick to good orthopedic principles. Your patient is a competitive athlete for a relative short portion of his or her life. Think about the long-term consequences of your treatment. Do not let coaches influence your judgment on treatment or return to play. Take time to talk to your young athletes' parents, even if doing so means calling them long distance after work.

Be a friend to your athletic trainers. They are overtrained, underpaid, and overworked. They do what they do because they love it. Enjoy working with your young athletes; they will be the joy of your practice!

–John F. Meyers, MD

Always remember that the athlete you treat, no matter at what level, is a patient. Therefore, you should discuss the diagnosis and treatment options and let the athlete decide what is best, just as you would for any other patient. The recent emphasis on confidentiality rules has made things easier in some ways; it is clear that we need the athlete's permission before disclosing information with coaches, administrators, owners, etc. In general, however, what is best for the athlete personally usually is what is best for the team in the long run.

–Ken Fine, MD

My one piece of advice would be to stay a bit detached from the team you are covering. By that I mean, if you are covering a collegiate or professional team, remember that your first responsibility is to the proper care of the athlete and not to the university, the parents, the team, or the ownership. There are certainly several stakeholders in any decision involving the athlete, but getting too close can sometimes compromise objectivity. Be a good communicator and keep in the loop the people that need to be there. Being a team orthopedist at any level has been incredibly rewarding for me, and it is always a privilege to participate.

–Dev K. Mishra, MD

The best advice I can give someone at any level is that you can't be a fan! You can enjoy the game and the competition, but you have to divorce yourself from getting emotionally involved in the outcome because becoming involved will cloud your judgment. At the end of the day, the only thing that matters is that you do what is best for the patient. Most participants won't remember who won the game, but everyone will remember if you do the wrong thing. It is becoming more difficult at every level of athletics because of the distrust between player and management. A team physician, although having to be sensitive to both points of view, must take all factors into consideration, but must do the RIGHT thing.

–John Xerogeanes, MD

Covering events and games is fun. Often you will find that you are one of the biggest fans of the team, but be careful not to allow the excitement to cloud your judgment. You are always the athlete's doctor first. Make decisions based purely on the best interest of the athlete in front of you. Problems happen when you let the portion of the season, impact of the game, or effect on the team or management interfere. When in doubt, treat the athlete as you would your own child.

–Mark Hutchinson, MD

A team physician is always on call. In private practice, you are (or should be) available at all hours. The same is true for a team physician. You must go to practices frequently and get to know the athletes personally. You must be present to assist coaches as to who is available and when he or she can compete. Doing so is essential because you are part of the team. In caring for high school teams, remember that the player may be from a family in an HMO. Although you may have the trust of the player, family, and coach, the HMO makes the decision as to treatment, especially surgery, and it may not be you. This decision is a financial one and not directed at you. Cooperate with the HMO physician and all will benefit.

–George A. Snook, MD

With regard to high school football teams, remember that you are solely on the field for the players and the community. Before you take on a high school, realize that unlike the pros, where you deal primarily with the players and coaches, you are also dealing with Mom and Dad. Make sure that everyone understands the treatment goals. The worse thing to deal with is a mother who feels that her baby is being pushed back on the field too early. Finally, encourage players to go to other physicians if they or their family have a working relationship with another doctor. Make sure to communicate freely with that physician to update the coach on the player's status.

–Beau Sasser, MD

Get very comfortable with the "risk versus reward" equation; it applies at all levels of sports medicine and changes with every game. When in doubt, take less risk.

–T. O. Souryal, MD

Always be honest with yourself and the athlete. Our mission is to ensure that an athlete has the opportunity to play safely at his or her highest capability. This mission can result in the team physician making unpopular decisions to protect the athlete. Do not be afraid to upset the coaches, athletic directors, parents, and the athlete when you make a command decision to place the athlete's health and safety above winning a game or a championship.

—Albert D. Olszewski, MD

You must think of the long-term risks of participation when clearing an athlete to play. Coaches, agents, even parents may not be putting the best interests of the athlete first when deciding on fitness to play. It is often a lonely decision to hold an athlete from participation, but that is what you are there to do.

—Edward R. McDevitt, MD

Don't compromise the athlete's care for the sake of short-term gains. Educating the athlete and the coaches about the nature of the injury and the long-term implications can go a long way in gaining their confidence and compliance.

—Anonymous

Working as a successful team physician is a responsibility that requires years of activity and experience. Your number one priority should be the care and well being of the athlete. Success as a team physician requires clinical excellence combined with an ability to communicate with the entire organization, starting with the athletic trainer. Communication is the key, and it involves listening, not talking. My advice for the junior orthopedic surgeon is to start small and take advantage of any opportunity that comes your way. Take great care of your teams and have patience. My advice for the senior team physicians is to share: teach a junior person the art of being a successful team doc and share your success with him or her. Lastly, be pleasant at all times; the best orthopedic job in the world usually involves some aspect of athletic team care.

—Anonymous

Protect the patient/athlete from the wishes of parents, coaches, and vendors. Do the right thing. Think of the patient first, income and public recognition last. Stay with what you are good at, but keep an open mind for subtle gradual improvements in technique. Recognize your limits and learn the art of looking intelligent when you tell a patient that you may not know the answer to his or her problem. Have a list of intelligent colleagues with trustworthy judgment that may know the answer, and do not be too proud to refer.

Treat athletes like real people. Tissue heals at the same rate no matter how good a patient is in sports. An ACL graft is an ACL graft, and you can't make it heal more quickly. A concussion has the same implications no matter who is affected. Be a good doctor and avoid being led astray because you are a team doctor.

—Anonymous

Always do your best for the patient. Our obligations are always to the patient. No other secondary considerations should be taken into account in ultimate decision making. I have avoided situations with financial considerations.

I have volunteered my time to covering games. I have enjoyed treating athletes, so my office is always available to the student athletes of the schools with which I have special relationships. I want them to feel that they have easy access to great care. I also have cared for Olympic-level athletes (1994 and 2002 Winter Games). No matter what the level, it is with pride that I watch an athlete achieve a goal at the limit of his or her ability. Whether it is televised around the world or seen by a collective group of parents and friends, there is nothing better. Avoid special arrangements with sports agents. Their job is to look out for their athletes. They may seem like they want to work with you, but if your advice does not fit in their plans, watch out! They can be very vindictive.

−Mahlon Bradley, MD

Being a team physician is not the same thing as being the orthopedic surgeon for a team. Once you decide to become a team physician in your community, do everything you can to be exactly that—a physician, not solely a surgeon. Doing so involves a commitment to discuss medical areas of concern to your patient and spending time with your school's athletic trainer to help his or her management of student athletes; most notably, it requires you to become adept at managing sports injuries and not simply bone and joint problems.

−J. Randy Percy, MD

Never ask or expect to be compensated monetarily for your efforts as team physician at any level of sport. To do so is an ethical dilemma. You will be much more professionally satisfied by the services you provide in an unbiased manner.

−Len Remia, MD

There are two areas in which I want to offer advice. One, let the coaches and athletic training staff know from day one that you are conservative and always have the student athlete's best "medical interest" foremost in your mind and that you will never let a player return to the sport before he or she is ready. Two, it is beneficial to let the head coach know that you are proud to be part of the program and even to use the word "passionate" about your job. Most head coaches see themselves this way, and knowing that the team doc is on the same page is beneficial for everyone.

−Anonymous

Be firm and quiet, and clarify every aspect of the injury to the patients and to the athletic trainer. Keep the patient's safety foremost in your mind.

−Anonymous

Stay true to the principles of anatomy and physiology. Do not treat injuries emotionally; doing so might mean the end of a player's high school, college, or professional career. Do not be afraid to take a player out of a game for his or her safety. Do not give information to the media. Give information to a team representative only.

–David B. Wilson, MD

Understand that your role as a team physician may have contradictory responsibilities. Oftentimes, your enthusiasm to return a key player to competition may conflict with your ethical responsibility as a physician. Young team docs in particular may feel more pressure from parents, fans, coaches, other players, and team administrators. Decisions concerning treatment and return to play must be medically sound and ethically responsible; under these circumstances, should the athlete seek additional consultation, the team physician can rest assured that care has been clinically appropriate and morally just.

–Andrew L. Chen, MD

Don't ever pay to take care of a team. Take care of teams if you enjoy taking care of teams. If you are just looking for surgeries, consider writing, research, and development of surgical techniques as an alternative.

The athletic trainer is most important in effectively taking care of the patient and coordinating care. Involve internists, cardiologists, and other professionals as much as possible in high school physicals and make it a community activity, if possible.

–Heinz Hoenecke, MD

COMMUNICATION

My advice based on experience on the sidelines follows two principles: trust and communication. When a player comes off the field and needs to be assessed, the coaching staff needs to be given the heads-up if he or she is not immediately available. They need to be told that the player is being evaluated and that, until it is completed, they should substitute the position. When the physician and athletic trainer walk off and "disappear," the coaching staff can get irritated at not being informed. A simple heads-up as to the status is invaluable at relieving that tension and giving you time to do a complete assessment. If a player's parents are around, it is always best to inform them as well regarding the nature and severity of the problem. They feel like outsiders looking in, but they are very much a concerned party and should be kept in the loop.

That's the communication pearl. The trust part is simple. You must have a good working relationship with the coaching and training staff to allow you to make the call on return to play and not be second guessed. Often, your judgment will be undermined by assistant coaches or others who think that you may be needlessly keeping players out. All of a sudden you may find players being shuttled away and getting notes from other docs who said it is okay to play. This communication is not something that comes easily, but it is worth establishing and protecting.

–Kenneth Jurist, MD

Frequently, when we care for our athletes, it is in a clinic setting. Although this scenario is fine for weekly follow-up evaluations, it is important to spend time with the athlete away from the other players when discussing significant issues. Players deserve the same privacy as other patients. This principle is especially true when you are planning to proceed with surgery, and it will allow the player to discuss all the issues pertaining to his or her injury without the stress of being around the other players and staff. This point may be minor, but although players are members of teams, their privacy should be respected.

–Christopher C. Annunziata, MD

In my years of experience as a team physician, I have found that the most important component to success is communication. Communication with a single voice and consistent message to the athletic trainer, athlete, and head coach or general manager is paramount. Make certain that each understands on his or her level the significance, recommended treatment options, and time to return to play for any injury. Always be honest and straightforward in communication, with the best interest of the athlete in mind. Remember, we are clinicians, not politicians.

–Scott Gillogly, MD

Within HIPAA guidelines, the team physician should communicate information regarding the health status of an athlete directly to both the certified athletic trainer and head coach in a timely fashion. Misinformation can be a frequent cause of mismanagement, unnecessary confusion, and stress. When dealing with adolescents, parents should also be included in this process.

–Peter A. Indelicato, MD

Having open, direct lines of communication with the training staff is vital to the quality of care of the athlete at any level. Establish early who communicates with the coaching staff or management. It should be ONE person only, so that they do not get two different stories as to time out or playing status. This procedure ensures that everyone is on the same page. Also, I highly recommend that you absolutely refuse to speak to the media regarding injuries, which will eliminate you as the responsible party for anything appearing in the media that the team does not want made public. You may explain about the injury to the person who is responsible for reporting to the media, but let that individual decide what to disclose to the media.

–Brian Crites, MD

When you are offering an opinion on the injury or condition of a player, particularly a critical player, to coaching staff, it is crucial to be as definitive as possible and use the most basic wording possible to explain the condition. As physicians, we are in the practice of using data, literature, and experience to validate and back up our opinion. Coaches rely on players for their livelihood and need to make decisions based on our recommendations. It is important to explain that a player has a "three-ligament knee injury" rather than an ACL/partial PCL/MCL injury, for example. Using basic language helps them to understand the difference between this injury and a simple ACL tear or "one-ligament knee injury" in terms of expectations for recovery and return to play following surgery.

–Michael J. Battaglia, II, MD

Don't deal directly with any of the management on the team, except the training staff. Always make sure that the entire medical staff, as well as the training staff, is on the same "page" when discussing medical issues with a player. Never discuss one player's medical situation with another player on the team.

–Peter MacDonald, MD

Inform all patients that every surgical procedure might have complications. Before operation acceptance, all patients have to consider whether the advantages of the operation outweigh the risks.

–Somsak Kuptniratsaikul, MD

It seems to be very helpful to use someone who knows the athletic trainers and coaches (ex-coaches or ex-athletic trainers are ideal) in the area to serve as a liaison, which will help open lines of communication that would otherwise not even be present.

–Anonymous

With respect to media relations, be aware of potential pitfalls that can possibly place you under increased litigious exposure, in spite of the allure of being involved with media. Consider carefully discussions about player injuries to members of the media, especially in light of HIPAA regulations.

–Anonymous

When it comes to caring for college-level athletes, keep all lines of communication open among your partners who may help with your team coverage, the team athletic trainers, the therapist, the coaching staff, and the injured athletes. Doing so will keep the entire health care organization on the same sheet of music and speaking with one voice. Nobody likes working in an information vacuum.

–LTC Tom DeBerardino, MD

Availability and good communication are the most important components of treating athletes. The team physician should explain the injury, recovery, surgery, and likelihood of returning to competition to the athlete, involved family (parents, significant other), athletic trainer, and coach. The physician should be available at all times via cell phone or pager to answer questions or address concerns or new injuries. Good communication and physician availability instill confidence in the athletes, families, and training and coaching staffs.

—Robin West, MD

It is vitally important that everyone understands his or her role, ie, the physician makes the medical decisions regarding the athletic injuries, not the sporting staff. Likewise, the athletic trainer(s) must be an extension of the physician. The coaching staff may have input regarding their needs with a given player but not in making the decision whether to play. Also, when a player returns, having been cared for by another physician, even if "cleared to play," the team physician should always have the final decision as to whether that player may return to action. During the rehabilitation of that individual, if the treating doctor is in the same city, I would also insist that the athlete's personal doctor guide that rehabilitation. That way, the player cannot try to "manipulate" his or her care between two physicians. Communication between all treating physicians is helpful in preventing this sort of problem.

—Graham Johnstone, MD

INTERACTIONS WITH ATHLETIC TRAINERS AND PHYSICAL THERAPISTS

In high school and college sports, a good, honest relationship with your athletic trainers is a must. You must know early on the capabilities of the athletic trainers, what they can do well, where they are weak, how to best communicate with them, how they handle the training room, how effective they are with the coaches and athletic directors, and what they want of you. This knowledge can be used to build a working relationship that will best fit your needs and the athletic trainer's responsibilities. Use the athletic trainer to help you with the day-to-day details. The athletic trainer can smooth out relationships with the coaches and athletic directors, communicate with the players more frequently, prepare the athletes for your advice, and implement things you can't do. You need to be prospective with the athletic trainer in deciding how to handle the tough calls, including decisions on return to or removal from play.

—W. Kibler, MD

Develop a good working relationship with the athletic trainers caring for the teams you cover. Always treat them with respect, as professionals and as critical members of the team, no matter what level of athletic competition you are covering. Additionally, get to know your patients' therapists. Send detailed postoperative instructions for therapy—don't assume that they know your protocol or that the protocol they have on file is acceptable for your patients without reviewing it first. Answer their phone calls.

—Anonymous

As all athletes and team physicians know, the team athletic trainer is the medical provider most closely tied to the players. All injuries, rehab, and care of the athletes funnel through the athletic trainer in both directions. He or she gains the athlete's trust and correctly controls their care. Failing to realize this phenomenon can lessen a team physician's effectiveness and worth significantly. Although it is sometimes difficult to determine, the amount of input and care a physician provides revolves around the relationship with the athletic trainer. If an athletic trainer believes in you and trusts that you care for the well-being of the athletes, the time spent on the field and in the training room will be rewarding and effective.

—Anonymous

Recognize that the athletic trainers can be your best ally or your worst adversary. They deal with athletes on a daily basis and have great influence on them. They can direct an athlete to seek consultation or even surgery from a particular physician (especially in a college situation in which there may be several physicians covering athletes) and influence whether the athlete seeks a second opinion. Therefore, treat the athletic trainers with the respect that they are due, and keep them in the loop regarding treatment decisions and dealings with the athletes. If you respect them, they will respect you.

—Christina Allen, MD

The athletic trainer is your best friend—never blow him off. Have a "sit down" with the coaches of the teams so that everyone knows your aims. You should make the injury or play decisions. Remember, no injury is minor to the player or coach; all deserve some attention. If asked by a player if he or she may have a second opinion, the answer is yes. Otherwise, the player and coach will think that you are hiding something. Most of these individuals at the college or high school level will accept your decisions. It may be different in the pro situation, depending on your reputation. However, no matter how great an athlete you were, you are a doc now. They are not interested in your 90-yard run against Cathedrale High. Later, it may come out that you played, and you may get silent kudos.

In college, 50% of the athletes are female. You had better be sure that you understand that fact and that they deserve the same care as male athletes.

Work out with the athletics director, owner, and coach exactly what you can say to the press. The less, the better. One careless quote can ruin a career.

—Robert Leach, MD

Never insult the athletic trainers or disagree with them in front of other people. Take it to the back room or office, but never make the athletic trainers look bad.

—Anonymous

The athletic trainer is your key to success. If you have a bad relationship with an athletic trainer, it will result in a bad experience for you and adversely affect your ability to take care of athletes effectively both in and out of the training room. A little humility and honest friendship goes a long way.

–Mark D. Miller, MD

Although you may have the most sports medicine knowledge of those that you work with in a given sports medicine arena, always respect the knowledge and opinions of the athletic trainers, physical therapists, students, chiropractors, massage therapists, and other health care workers. These people are hardworking professionals or professionals-in-training, and they deserve common courtesy. Such courtesy engenders their respect, and it is the proper way to treat people. They will be your advocates with coaches, athletes, and athletes' families. Superseding all else, always make sure the any care given is in the best interest of every athlete.

–Randy Schwartzberg, MD

Respect the skill, experience, and training of each member of the sports medicine team. As a sports medicine–trained orthopedic surgeon, you probably don't know the best way to tape an ankle, rehab a hamstring injury, or condition a postinjury athlete. Most failures in the efficient management of injured athletes occur because of communication failures. Make yourself easily available to the other members of your team (athletic trainers) and speak to them with respect and professionalism. They have earned their position, just as you have yours.

Surround yourself with good doctors. You will never be the expert at everything. Don't imply that you are. Be good at what you do and be the "go-to guy" for everything in orthopedic sports medicine. Be equipped with a team of good physicians to whom you happily refer those conditions for which you are not the expert (eg, hand surgery, spine, general surgery, eye, general medicine).

The goal is to get the athlete better and back on the field. Nowhere does it say that you are the one who needs to do everything, but respect for you will be enhanced if you can, as team physician, facilitate the process, whether you are the actual provider of care or refer the athlete to someone else who provides care.

When you are successful, give, or at the very least share, the credit with the athletic trainers. They work very hard and are seriously underpaid. They deserve recognition that they often don't get. Take your own credit in the way you feel when what you did helped someone else to succeed.

–Kirt M. Kimball, MD

Respect the athletic trainers. They are well-trained, usually very conscientious, and often have knowledge you might not, especially in areas outside of our specialty. My temptation is to feel that, as the doctor, I should have all the answers, which of course I can't. Using their input not only may result in better treatment of an injured athlete, but also creates a sense of teamwork and fellowship that can be valuable when challenges arise.

                                                                    —Thomas Merchant, MD

Beware of well-meaning physical therapists who want to treat everyone like they are 18 years old. Although most physical therapists realize that the treatment should be customized to the patient, there are some who do not have expertise at rehabilitating sports injuries. Without experience, they may be just fine for a 75-year-old hip fracture, but that doesn't mean they will have the expertise to handle an ACL protocol. It is important to know your therapists and communicate your protocol with them. Have open lines of communication with the therapists and with the athletic trainers so that they know the factors that will influence the rehabilitation.

                                                                              —Anonymous

DEALING WITH OTHER DOCTORS AND SECOND OPINIONS

If you don't know something about an injury or condition, admit it and find someone who does know. Don't ever hesitate to refer to someone else something that is outside your expertise or field, and don't get upset when athletes get second or third opinions. If a player is really upset by one of your decisions, make sure the decision is not made in a vacuum. Seek the advice of the athletic trainer, and, if necessary, the coaches, although the latter may have their own agenda. In these cases, second opinions from people you trust often are helpful. An opinion from doctors you do not know is fine, too, but it is best to get the most knowledgeable people in either case.

                                                                 —Edward G. McFarland, MD

If you go to a practice where a senior partner is taking care of the athletic teams, make sure that you are not perceived by that partner as a threat, which can lead to all sorts of nastiness. Not only will the partner potentially withdraw and not support you, but it also can make the others involved with the team unsure and uneasy.

                                                                              —Anonymous

When your health care system decides to contribute to a team and asks you to be the team physician, it is probably fine. However, it is not appropriate for you personally to pay for the privilege of taking care of the team.

                                                                              —Anonymous

Tell the players at the beginning of the season that you do not mind if they get second opinions. However, encourage them not to go out on their own to get it. You may be able to get them seen by someone who is more qualified than they would choose on their own. For example, in the case of a head injury, the player may seek a second opinion by his or her family doctor or a neurologist with no background in sports medicine and be told that he or she is out for the entire season or career. However, if the player saw someone else, he or she may be able to come back SAFELY at a sooner date.

–Brian Crites, MD

If your athlete goes to see a physician who does what you do for a living and is going to see that physician because he or she is famous or has a "big name," do not worry about it. Most physicians are busy enough without worrying about this sort of thing. Also, the "big name" gets to live with the good results and bad results, just like you do.

–Anonymous

Although taking care of a high-profile team can get patients in the door, you will lose players to outside doctors in the end if you don't have a team of specialists that work with you to treat all the types of injuries that occur. Taking care of a high-level team is good for your ego early in your career, but the liability involved and the lack of long-term patient referrals isn't worth it. You are much better off taking care of a local college, but make sure that you have the players see the best person possible for their problems, and don't try to treat every problem yourself. Be low key but available to make sure each athlete gets the best possible care.

–Anonymous

When treating college students from out of town, do not hesitate to get doctors in the students' hometown involved with care. Just because you are the team doctor doesn't mean the athlete can't or shouldn't be treated where his or her family may be more comfortable with the physician. Being flexible to assist with preoperative or postoperative care can be as worthwhile to the student athlete and the athletic trainers as performing the surgery.

–Jonathan Krome, MD

If you get other physicians involved in taking care of the teams with you, be gracious, but let them know that you are in charge and that they should not undermine your relationship with the hierarchy. Be wary if your partner begins to come forward with information from the athletic director, athletic trainers, or coaches that you do not have.

–Anonymous

Work closely with others whose advice you respect. When taking care of high-level athletes (and ALL patients, for that matter), a partner with whom you can discuss cases and perform complicated surgical procedures, and from whom you can obtain second opinions, is invaluable. Such a partnership is both personally satisfying (ie, builds relationships and camaraderie) and professionally conscientious (especially if an athlete has a less than satisfactory outcome from your intervention).

–Brett Wasserlauf, MD

OTHER POINTERS AND ADVICE

If you accept the responsibility of covering for a team, be aware that it often entails caring for the visiting team as well. Show up on time, which includes warm-up as well as the game. In one situation, my hockey team was the visiting team, and during warm-up, the goalie got struck in the neck with a puck and went into laryngospasm. The home team physician was nowhere to be found. The athletic trainer established an airway and avoided a very nasty situation both for the goalie and the team doctor who was responsible.

–Robert P. Mack, MD

Identify all of the other health folks at an event: EMTs, paramedics, athletic trainers, other docs. Introduce yourself and find out how the others want to handle certain things. Find out where the nearest hospital is and what level of trauma care it provides, especially in a foreign country. Don't be so insecure that you cannot look up something with which you are not familiar. Have back-up colleagues to call and Internet access. The coach needs accurate, specific data. He or she needs to know if and when a player will be ready to play. Give realistic, not optimistic or pessimistic, expectations.

–Peter Gerbino, MD

Prepare properly for the injuries that will occur not only in games but also in practice. Conduct a drill each season with athletic trainers and coaches to practice safely moving an athlete with a possible spinal cord injury. Your athletes will be tempted by performance-enhancing drugs. Do not facilitate their use. Even if all your opponents are cheating, help your athletes compete using the best legal training advances available. Keep learning.

–Edward R. McDevitt, MD

Serious, catastrophic, and life-threatening injuries rarely occur, but you always must anticipate the worst. A cardiac emergency is more likely to occur in a spectator, such as a parent or grandparent, than in a player. However, formulate a plan for resuscitation and emergency transport before the event:

- Introduce yourself to the ambulance crew (if available onsite).
- Establish a means of communication with the hospital or ambulance company: cell phone or determine phone location if there is no cell service.
- Identify potential help in attendance (athletic trainer, physician, EMT, nurse, student, coach).

- Start with the ABCs of basic cardiopulmonary resuscitation by establishing responsiveness and initiating treatment as necessary, but prompt transport to a hospital is the key.

—Mike Stuart, MD

Get to know the sport you are taking care of and its technical rules as soon as possible! Also, get to know the administrators of the sport.

—R. T. Herrick, MD

Know the medicolegal parameters of your team or event coverage. Will you be responsible for the actions of all school personnel? What about follow-up off the field (eg, concussion, compartment syndrome)? Who has the say on return to sports? Know the medical history of the players. Go over these with the athletic trainer or coach. Get to the game ahead of time and don't miss the first play or the last. Make sure you have the authority to stop the game or prevent a player from returning.

The level of decision making can vary with the level of sport. That which might be done in the pros is not appropriate in a high school or youth league. Lack of immediate radiographic assessment or adequate athletic trainer support will limit return to play. There is no room for presumptive diagnosis. Although I have heard colleagues say that they would reduce a dislocation on the field, I disagree. It is important to substantiate the injury and any occult fracture before definitive treatment. Splint them where they lie; when in doubt, ship them out. An exception would be obvious vascular compromise.

To understand what we know and don't know is true knowledge. It is important to avoid snap diagnoses, to consider the complete differential diagnosis of the symptoms, and to consider the risks. When approaching an injured player, observe, question, palpate, and do functional tests.

Remember, there is no instant replay for community play. Watch the game; the moment of injury reveals the mechanism as well as the potential for damage. The following are actual examples. (1) A kid gets a hard block to his left flank by a much more physical player; he can't return immediately because of pain. Later he is noted to have a prominent skin bruise over his kidney area and splenic area, and despite these findings he is allowed to go home. Later, he presents in the emergency room with a splenic hematoma and hematuria. (2) A soccer player is kicked in the shin so hard that he drops on the field, limps off, and does not return. He is allowed to ride a bicycle home. Later, he presents with a compartment syndrome associated with a nondisplaced midshaft tibial fracture.

—Wayne B. Leadbetter, MD

When doing preparticipation physicals for minor league baseball, especially independent ball, the athletes should be dressed in shorts only. Players don't want to tell you about previous surgeries because they want to make the team. You have to look for arthroscopy scars and carefully evaluate wrists, elbows, shoulders, and knees. Athletes will try to deny problems early and then admit to them during the season. Get records if you have questions.

–Juliet DeCampos, MD

At away games, you may not have privileges at the local hospital, so clarify with the home team's physician who will be caring for any of your injured players needing to go to the local hospital. In turn, assure your visiting physicians and athletic trainers that you will be supervising the care of their injured players. Although it may be rare, you might consider staying overnight with the injured players because they, their family, your athletic trainers, and the coaches will need you to communicate what is happening to the injured players at that time. Although you may not have privileges at the local hospital, your input into any medical decision-making processes will be invaluable and will provide all of the aforementioned people a sense of knowing that their physician is involved in caring for the injured athlete.

–Robert S. Burger, MD

Insist on having your team's players complete detailed medical and orthopedic history forms before each season. This information, along with preseason physical examinations, goes a long way in providing the best service to your players. As orthopedic surgeons covering athletic events, it is imperative that we understand and are aware of the nonorthopedic medical conditions that can afflict our players, such as type 1 diabetes or exercise-induced bronchospasm. In addition, as the level of competition reaches that of the professional athlete, history and physical examination documents become paramount for player contract purposes and potentially for medicolegal reasons.

–Kyle Flik, MD

Clin Sports Med 26 (2007) 285–304

CLINICS IN SPORTS MEDICINE

EVIER
NDERS

Trends for the Future as a Team Physician: Herodicus to Hereafter

James Whiteside, MD[a], James R. Andrews, MD[b],*

[a]400 University Park Drive, Apartment 381, Birmingham, AL 35209, USA
[b]Alabama Sports Medicine & Orthopaedic Center, 806 St. Vincent's Drive, Suite 415,
Birmingham, AL 35205, USA

Much has transpired in the world of sports medicine since Herodicus [1], a Thracian physician of the fifth century BC, rendered his foundational theories on the use of therapeutic exercise for the maintenance of health and the treatment of disease. Unfortunately, as basic knowledge advances, history abounds in inconsistencies in regard to the proper and most effective delivery of sports medicine. One additional truth that must be added to the human equation of the established facts of death and taxes is the realization that sports participation does produce injuries, some of which are severe, career-ending, and even deadly.

In 1890 at Harvard University [2] in Cambridge, Massachusetts it became apparent that unattended, uncoached, and academically unsupervised team sports activities frequently produced significantly large numbers of musculoskeletal injuries. In order for team sports activities to be of benefit personally and to society, the reduction of the frequency and severity of injuries in team sports became paramount. As a consequence, a program was instituted to educate the players of a sport as to the need for personal fitness, the use of proper gear, the need for treatment of all injuries, and the importance of rehabilitation. The athlete was expected as a student gentleman to act prudently. Coaches were hired and assigned to a sport, and properly informed as to team preparation, exercise, conditioning, and the awareness of the need for immediate care of all injuries. Trainers and the therapists were expected to follow standard methods of rehabilitation and to facilitate early return to full activity. The athletic department was responsible for the supervision of the team program, and for providing proper facilities, rehabilitation, personnel, and equipment as well as scheduling of games. That same year, the team physician [2] was recognized and designated as the team surgeon. He was charged with the full responsibility for the care and health of the athletes and with striving to prevent injuries.

*Corresponding author. *E-mail address*: james.andrews@asmoc.com (J.R. Andrews).

0278-5919/07/$ – see front matter
doi:10.1016/j.csm.2007.01.009
© 2007 Published by Elsevier Inc.
sportsmed.theclinics.com

This progressive type of sports medicine team approach met with only minimal criticism from the misinformed, and proved to be quite successful, as carefully collected records indicated. Many of the larger Eastern universities successfully used comparable programs. Smaller universities and secondary schools continued in the previous methodology, primarily because of lack of motivated personnel.

Dr. Darling [3] was given credit for publishing in 1899 the earliest scientific report on the physiologic effects of strenuous athletic endeavors within this new team approach to aid in decreasing the injury rate. Also, Dr. Darling emphasized the need for medical supervision of the athletes.

As reported by Nichols and Richardson [4], in 1904, the year Helen Keller was born, Dr. Nichols, as football team surgeon, changed football rules so that it became mandatory to report all injuries, and to wear head gear, shoulder, and thigh pads, and "braced" shoes. A carefully compiled injury record collected from 1904 to 1905 revealed a significant decrease in injuries sustained in football [5].

The death of 20 on-the-field football players in 1905 caused President Theodore Roosevelt to form the American Football Rules Committee to establish new safety precautions that would embrace the forward pass [6]. One member of that committee was Henry L. Williams, MD, who had been a star halfback at Yale and who later coached and was Athletic Director at the University of Minnesota. The work of this committee led to the formation of the National Collegiate Athletic Association (NCAA) in 1910 [7].

In 1925, a new, well-equipped medical facility was completed at Harvard. In addition to deep heat modalities and whirlpool baths, a radiograph department was installed, and three physical therapists were hired. Also in 1925, for the first time the medical department made an attempt to follow the injured athlete through the academic year or until discharged symptom-free.

A dietician to supervise all training tables was instituted in 1927 [2], and as a result, gastrointestinal upsets decreased appreciably. Incidentally, the dietitian noted that football and crew athletes required twice the number of calories per day when compared with players of non-contact sports.

In Germany in the years before and after World War I, there was a renewed impetus in sports medicine [8]. The Germans were the first to use the term "sports physicians" in 1904, and they held a sports physicians congress in 1912, the year the Titanic went down. This evolved into the German Association of Sports Physicians. At St. Moritz, Switzerland in 1920, German leadership led to discussions with Olympic dignitaries that ultimately produced the formation of an international sports medicine organization, Association International Medico-Sportive (AIMS) [9]. Its purpose was to promote clinical and scientific research in cooperation with sports federations and to meet at Olympic sites. This organization became FIMS in 1933 (Federation Internationale de Medico-Sportive et Cientifique). In Berlin in 1936, the year Jessie Owens' victories ruined the day for Hitler, 1500 physicians from 40 countries attended the FIMS meeting. Unfortunately, few Americans availed themselves of this or other earlier meetings. Herxheimer [10], a German physician whose publication was translated and retitled "The Principles of Medicine in Sports for Physicians and Students," was noted to be quite influential, especially in Europe.

In 1932 Dr. Thorndike was named team surgeon at Harvard [2]. He instituted daily medical room coverage by the team surgeon. Also, he mandated that all body-contact team sports participants, whether at practice or at a game, have the services of the surgeon or physical therapist. At the insistence of colleague Dr. Arlie V. Bock, Dr. Thorndike assembled his experiences, knowledge, and review of pertinent literature into a monograph, *Athletic Injuries, Prevention, Diagnosis and Treatment,* that was first published in 1938 by Lea and Febiger and was followed by five revisions. This text served as a primary, practical source of pertinent information for all of the members of the sports medicine team well into the 1960s.

In the pre-World War II years, monumental contributions to the knowledge base of the physiology of the musculoskeletal system enabled sports physicians to care for the athlete with fact-based techniques, to establish physical fitness boundaries, and to instill injury preventive measure with confidence.

The Eggletons [11], Fiske and Subbarow [12], and Hill [13] were instrumental in introducing the concept of energy and heat production from the chemical breakdown of phosphocreatin and glycogen to advance from potential to musculoskeletal kinetic activity. Talbott and Michaelson [14] observed that heat cramps also occurred from salt loss and when exercise-induced body heat is not dissipated by sweating. In order to prevent heat cramps, Dill showed that when excessive salt is lost by sweating, the kidneys shut down salt excretion [15]. This pertinent study was gleaned from experience when building Boulder Dam and from workers at the Youngstown Steel Mill. It was not until 1945 that Ladell [16] reported sweat rates in excess of three liters per hour in conditions of heavy work in hot, humid weather. Studies in the Harvard Fatigue Laboratory by Edwards and Wood [17] noted leukocytosis with exercise incurred in a football game. Incidentally, Wood was the captain of the football team at that time. Hill and colleagues [18] studied lactic acid and oxygen consumption (debt) after exercise. In 1935, Edwards and colleagues [19] noted the fact that football players required 5000 to 6000 calories per day.

Anatomical publications in this same period revealed an interest in recurrent shoulder dislocations and their pathology, the etiology of elbow pain, and the remedy for knee meniscus injury. In 1938, Dr. Bankart [20] described a glenoid lesion that continues to bear his name. In 1936, Cyriax [21] described the diagnosis and treatment of tennis elbow. Also in 1936, Simon [22], in an article on the semilunar cartilage of the football knee, advocated removal of the entire injured meniscus. This methodology proved to be clinically beneficial initially, but most deleterious years later.

In 1930, Dill and colleagues [15] used a motor-driven, horizontal treadmill task for 20 minutes and then drew blood to check for lactic acid and carbon dioxide capacity. They determined that well-trained athletes performed much better, as demonstrated by their graphs. The treadmill still retains its status as foundational equipment in exercise gyms and training rooms.

An early, accurate test for fitness was developed by Johnson and colleagues [23] and published in 1942. The test was the 20-inch step test in rhythm for 5 minutes. Positive merit has proven the test to be worthy and it continues to be widely used. "The athletic heart is non-existent" stated H.L. Smith of the Mayo Clinic in Rochester, Minnesota, as quoted by Thorndike [2]. Cardiologists may tend to modify that pronouncement.

In 1947, the Baruch Committee on Physical Medicine formed a subcommittee to define physical fitness. In essence, the report stated that physical fitness is a functional concept rather than a anatomic one, and that more data were needed on physical capacity and physiological adjustment. The ambiguity of that report fails to recognize the pioneer efforts of Edward Hitchcock [24], who as a college physician at Amherst College in the 1880s and 1890s developed a system of physical fitness exercises that served as the basic model for physical education (PE) for American schools and colleges. Dr. Hitchcock, a Harvard graduate and an avid anthropometrician, believed that a sound mind and physical fitness produced productivity.

Doping in sports is ancient and certainly not a new phenomenon. In 1941, Hellebrandt and Karpovich [25] reviewed the use of artificial stimulants (common in horse and dog racing for many prior years) to allay fatigue. Many substances proved to be ineffective, with the exceptions of alcohol, amphetamine, coca leaves, and caffeine. Independently, Hellebrandt stated that caffeine delays the onset of fatigue.

In an attempt to further reduce injury in sport, in 1957 Quigley [26] produced the individual athlete's Bill of Rights. The bill called for good coaching, good equipment, and good medical care, which includes preseason examination and presence at every practice or game. Unfortunately, this bill has lacked full compliance.

Not only have care, treatment, and management of athletic injuries improved, but also the interest in and application of the knowledge of nutrition has gained popularity. Dietary fat has been reduced, and an increase in carbohydrate consumption is used for endurance performance. Total calories, not testosterone, need to be increased for Tour de France cyclists

Proper training of athletes after World War II was deficient in a scientific basis for exercise physiology, factual knowledge, and experimental investigation. In 1948, Schneider and Karpovich [27] published *Physiology of Muscular Activity*, which provided an excellent fundamental insight into muscle performance.

In order for the sports physician to expertly prescribe an individual athletic training regimen that would maximize potential, evaluate progress and be relatively safe, fitness by strengthening as well as determination of aerobic capacity needed to be established. In 1951, Cureton [28] pioneered both strength and VO-2 max testing to evaluate and prescribe training programs. Delorme and Watkins [29] fostered progressive resistance exercises in 1948.

In the period after World War II, orthopedists Dutoit and Ensilin [30] performed a series of arthrotomies for internal derangement of the knee to establish a clinical diagnosis. Originally invented by Hey of Leeds in England in

1782 [31], the term "internal derangement" also was noted to be uncertain and confusing. In 1945, Pendergrass and Lafferty [32], established the radiographic finding of widening of the space between the distal tibia, fibula, and calcaneous in significant ankle injuries. An interpretation of this radiograph is termed a mortis view and remains standard today. In an article published in 1947 with regard to the fixation of acromioclavicular separation, Dr. Bosworth [33] proposed a screw approximation. Unfortunately, the fixation prevented functional clavicular rotation. Bennett [34], in a study of shoulders and elbows of pitchers published in 1947, remarked on the frequent finding of a lesion on the inferior margin of the glenoid usually found in curve-ball pitchers. The etiology was assumed to be caused by traction on the origin of the triceps. A recent review article by Andrews and colleagues [35] reveals newer orthopedic data on the formation of the Bennett's lesion.

In 1947, the clinical field of treatment of infection was addressed by Dr. Keefer [36] for treatment of furuncles, impetigo, and open wounds with daily injection of 600,000 units of penicillin in beeswax and peanut oil. Staphylococcus/streptococcus infections often were grouped together and treated alike.

After World War II, America was exuberant and vigorous and life was good. Sports activity again acquired an elevated place in society. Team and individual sports were emphasized in elementary and high schools. A need for care of the athlete became obvious. As a consequence, local physicians simply volunteered or seemingly were just pressed into community service. Many who were generalists became identified with local schools and communities and provided care without compensation.

There was an insufficient amount of information available on sports medicine during those years. As a result, the generalist tended to rely on previous experience, military service, or just applied good medical judgment. Referrals to the orthopedist and other specialists increased overall acumen and enhanced the level of care for the athletes.

Also in the late 1940s and early 1950s, orthopedic team physicians, singly or as a group, aligned themselves with major universities by contract or at the pleasure of the administration or the coaches. Some orthopedists continued their long-time relationship with high schools and colleges as a service. A few orthopedic groups, to solidify their relationship and prestige with certain universities, were alleged to have endorsed scholarships at those schools.

About 1950, a totally new appearance of sports medicine sideline coverage came upon the scene. This type of coverage ranged from a single individual attempting to care for a team all the way to an orthopedic group that would "cover" several high schools as well as colleges. Dr. Hughston [37] and his orthopedic group had covered local high schools in the Columbus, Georgia area and he personally serviced Auburn University in Auburn, Alabama. After some state resistance, Dr. Hughston's plan evolved into coverage of Friday night regional football games with trainers or physical therapists from his clinic, in concert and cooperation with the local schools' team physician. In addition, the trainer/physical therapist would visit the schools once or twice per week, establish rapport with the administration and the coaches, examine any injured athletes, suggest rehabilitation techniques, and advise orthopedic consultation when deemed necessary. It was customary for Dr. Hughston and his orthopedic group to be on the high school sidelines Friday night and at the college games on Saturday. This trend from disconnected, individual sports medicine care to a planned, consistent "outreach" approach with a central orthopedic backup proved to be quite efficient and successful. By 1959, similar outreach programs spread across Georgia to Alabama. Dr. Fred L. Allman, who played at the University of Georgia in Athens, had a similar affiliation with Georgia Tech in Atlanta and developed an outreach program to care for high school athletes from Atlanta and the surrounding area. Likewise, Dr. E.C. Brock enjoyed a very close relationship with the University of Alabama's coach Bryant and local athletes. Within a few years, Dr. William G. Clancy, Jr. at the University of Wisconsin in Madison, and Dr. Don H. O'Donoghue at the University of Oklahoma in Norman gave of their expertise for many years to athletes in their areas.

Two articles regarding the shoulder in this time period need mentioning. In 1951, Brav and Gulledge [38] discussed the Putti-Platt procedure for the treatment of anterior instability of the glenohumeral joint. In spite of the fact that the surgical result significantly limited the throwing motion, the operation largely was successful in preventing anterior subluxation. When the procedure was too tight, posterior shoulder symptoms resulted. Although used until the 1970s, the procedure was replaced by the Bristow, as described by Helfet [39] in 1958.

In 1959, McLaughlin [40] published a study on lesions of the rotator cuff. He described calcification in the subacromial bursa in the musculotendinous cuff. In an article from 1960 in the American Academy of Orthopaedic Surgeons (AAOS) Instructional Course, Quigley [41] suggested that a scaphoid fracture be casted for 12 weeks to obtain healing. Screw fixation was years away.

In a 1960 article in *Clinical Orthopedics and Related Research*, Thompson and colleagues [42] discussed the use and effectiveness of anti-inflammatory agents such as amylase, trypsin, and streptokinase in buccal form. Incidentally, streptokinase was administered to author Whiteside intravenously as an emergency procedure in 1988, for coronary artery occlusion. Also, Thompson and coworkers mentioned hyalouronidase, a form of which is now available for intrasynovial administration.

Probably the most influential article in that era concerning coma and serious and fatal head injury evaluation was written in 1961 by Schneider and colleagues [43]. That group analyzed fatal cases, discussed etiology, and outlined improvement in protective gear and technique. The same year, Rose and colleagues [44] at the University of Nebraska in Lincoln recommended the use of a pre-game liquid meal. Sustagen was the GatorPro of its day. It wasn't until 1967 that the *Journal of the American Dental Association* [45] announced the availability by its members to form a custom-fitted mouth protection (mouthpiece).

An outreach program emanating from an orthopedic group, a generalist group, or a university, is dependent upon the availability of athletic trainers, and their ability, training, and devotion to the athlete. Although generally recognized as an entity in 1938, the group was disbanded during World War II and reorganized as the National Athletic Trainers Association (NATA) in 1950. The NATA continues to enjoy a close affiliation with major orthopedic clinics as well as clinical centers.

Primarily as a result of Dr. Hughston's efforts as chairman of the Sports Medicine Committee of the American Orthopaedic Society, and the multiplicity of sports medicine conferences, there came about an abundance of sports medicine topics that needed to be published. The *Journal of Sports Medicine* was born in 1972, and later became the *American Journal of Sports Medicine*. It was soon realized that there was a need to further refine the orthopedic surgeon's skills in the field of sports medicine. This need was rectified by establishing an additional year of specialized training. The first orthopedic sports medicine fellowship was established in 1968, by Jack Wickstrom, MD at Tulane University in New Orleans, Louisiana [37]. Two years later, a similar fellowship was established at the Hughston Clinic in Columbus, Georgia. The first general sports medicine fellowships were started at the Hughston Clinic in 1984 and 1985 with Brian C. Halpern and the following year at the Cleveland Clinic in Ohio (1985–1986) with Rosemary Agostini.

After World War II, physical education was emphasized in elementary schools for both boys and girls. Girls began to play individual and team sports in high school and college. In 1972, Colleges and universities were required by law (Title IX) [46] to have an equal number of men and women teams and comparable resources. As a result, injury numbers increased, as did visits to the team physician, whose medical acumen and breath of knowledge were stressed.

Over the years, Olympic history reveals a female marathon runner in 1896 and females competing in tennis, archery, and swimming. Not until the 1984 Olympics [47] did women run all of the distance races. Medical examinations with gene identification became necessary after the 1964 Olympics [48] when two "women" were identified as men.

The 1970s brought a resurgence of interest in sports medicine. Considerable thought centered around the cause of ligamentous laxity after knee injury. Apparently, controversy fueled by lack of basic research, few patients, little follow-up surgery, and unorganized spread of pertinent information, resulted in failure to appreciate older orthopedic publications. Interest seemed to focus on anteromedial and arterolateral ligamentous laxity to explain and specifically treat knee instability [49–54]. It would appear that, as always, history is forgotten. The anterior cruciate ligament (ACL) as noted at times in early publications by Pringle [55] in 1907, Jones and Smith [56] in 1913, and by Alwyn Smith [57] in 1918, is referred to as the "crucial" ligament. Also, evidently, the ACL was known by Galen (circa 170 AD [58]). A significant hiatus of time elapsed before the rediscovery and study of the ACL occurred. In 1845, Bonnet [59] of Lyon described the clinical features of ACL rupture, including an audible crack, hemorrhage, and abnormal joint motion. This type of motion is now referred to as a positive Lachman test. The absence of resistance to anterior translation of the tibial on the femur, was reported by Noulis [60] in 1875, in deference to Dr. Torg and colleagues' statement [61].

Literature reveals that in 1895 Mayo Robson [62], was the first surgeon to repair a torn ACL. In 1920, Hey Groves [63] accurately described the abrupt, forward slipping of the tibia. The maneuver, as popularized by Drs. Hughston and Andrews [51,52] is known as the jerk test or the pivot shift of MacIntosh [64]. Replacement of the torn ACL by artificial material first was reported by Lange [65] of Munich in 1903, using silk sutures and the semitendinous tendon (ST). In 1914, Corner [66] used silver wire and in 1918, Alwyn Smith [57] used eight-ply, number 3 silk fixed to bone with bronzed wire. In 1927, Ludloff [67] augmented silk and fascia lata, as did Hey Groves. Since that time, other materials have served as ineffective substitutes for the torn ACL, such as nylon, Dacron, carbon fiber, polyproplene, polyester mesh, xenografts, kangaroo tendon, biceps aponeurosis, and even a meniscus. Galeazzi [68], after noting unfavorable outcomes of Hey Groves and Dupuy de Frenelle, published his techniques for reconstruction of the ACL using the semitendinosis (ST) tendon in 1934. Also, 1934 was the year when Dizzy Dean and brother Paul lost the World Series to Lefty Grove of the Detroit Tigers. Dizzy Dean also lost an exhibition game to Satchel Paige later in 1934.

After an interval of several years, a singular event ensued. In 1963, Jones [69] secured the too-short patella bone graft to the femur just anterior to the notch, using the central third of the patient's patellar tendon with the attached patellar bone block and with the distal end remaining attached. The results of the procedure proved to be only fair. In 1966, Bruckner [70] may have been the first to use the central third of the patellar tendon as a free graft.

Interestingly, there persisted a distinct difference of opinion as to the functional merit of the intact ACL. In 1935, Milch [71], stated that the ACL was not necessary. Also, Herzmark [72], in a 1938 publication, believed the ACL simply to be an embryological vestige of no worth. Conversely, Drs. Allman [73] in 1974 and Fetto and Marshall [74] in 1980 discussed the validity of ACL function in knee stability.

Because of the difficulty and, at times the impossibility of recognizing the pathology within the knee [75,76], visualization of the ACL and other soft tissue structures was deemed necessary to establish a more definitive diagnosis. This significant step forward was possible by the use of the radiograph and contrast arthrography. In 1921, Kleinberg [77] described the use of oxygen injected into the knee to perceive and discern soft tissue. Unfortunately, a case of air embolism dampened enthusiasm [78]. Pushing on, in 1938 Quaintance [79] published 50 successful cases of knee pneumo-radiography with confirmation by arthrotomy. Also, in 1938, Lindblom [80] described the appearance of knee ligaments by using contrast arthrography, which prompted the acceptance of the technology. With the development of soluble, urographic media, double-contrast techniques became well-established.

Investigation into the workings of the knee was enhanced by the use of a laparoscope for arthroendoscopy by Bircher [81] in 1921. A further report in 1922 stated that a torn meniscus diagnosis was confirmed in eight of nine of his cases by arthrotomy [82]. In 1925, Kreuscher [83] of Chicago was enthusiastic about his experience with the arthroscope that he designed. Cadaver studies in 1931 by Burman [84], from the Hospital for Joint Disease in New York, using an arthroscope, enabled him to visualize all the major joints. Finkelstein and Mayer [85] used the arthroscope to perform an intra-articular biopsy of the knee in 1931. Problems with optics, light sources, and gas/liquid media delayed common acceptance until the publication of an atlas by Watanabe and colleagues [86] of Japan in 1957, and the development of the No. 21 arthroscope, which combined fiber optics and a miniature television camera in 1972. After study in Japan, Drs. Jackson and Abe [87] came back to Canada and then to Baylor and popularized the technique. Dr. O'Connor [88] is given credit for performing the first partial minisectomy with the modified No. 21 scope.

There may have been favorable economics, a society that endorsed sports and the athlete, and the popularity of unique athletes and knowledge of their lifestyle and injuries, but a singular circumstance produced a dichotomy in the ranks of orthopedic surgeons. One group of orthopedists remained conventional, but the other group of orthopedists adopted the efficacy of the arthroscope. As a result, orthopedic sports medicine was reformulated.

Such a clear delineation, as noted in practicing orthopedists, does not exist, nor is there unification within those general sports medicine physicians. Petitioning the American Board of Medical Specialty Societies (ABMSS) to allow sports medicine as a specialty in the 1970s was not fruitful. The decision was based on the premise that those physicians who serve as medical team doctors represent multiple, diverse backgrounds. Yet during 1974, the ABMSS granted a specialty status to emergency physicians who are from varied professional backgrounds. Those emergency medicine examinations for board certification were begun in 1978, the last year a horse (Affirmed) won the Triple Crown for racing. At this writing, a certificate of added qualification (CAQ) examination is available for both orthopedic and medical team physicians.

In the 1970s and 1980s, a great number of general sports medicine physicians found employment or a close affiliation with NCAA-monitored colleges and universities. The team orthopedist remained assigned, but was less responsible for day-to-day care of the athletes. Sick call, observation, and control of athletic trainers/physical therapy activities, progression of rehabilitation/return to practice status, and communication with coaches while at daily practice would become the obligation of the medical team physician. This partial reversal of roles is analogous to child/parent reversal of roles in a family in which the child, now an adult, assumes precedence. Typically, the medical team physician has his or her office in the campus health center or its equivalent, whereas the orthopedic team physician maintains an office in the same area for one or two visits/examinations per week. Weekend coverage for football or other major sports remains unchanged. Also, the opinion of the orthopedist remains paramount and supersedes that of the medical team physician. In this scheme of things, the medical team physician must learn to play "second fiddle" expertly in order for this orchestra (medical team) to perform eloquently.

During this same period, postgraduate education for both the orthopedic and the medial team physician was available through conferences produced by the American College of Sports Medicine (ACSM), which was formed in 1954, the year Roger Bannister broke the 4-minute mile record. Also, the American Orthopedic Society for Sports Medicine (AOSSM), organized in 1972, offered courses and affiliate memberships for non-orthopedic physicians. The American Medical Society for Sports Medicine (AMSSM) was not formed until 1991.

The gold standard for reconstruction of the torn ACL was not yet achieved in the 1970s and early 1980s. In addition, there still existed the apparent need to control medial and lateral rotation. Newer techniques emerged. In 1976, Franke [89] published the first description using the middle one third of the patellar tendon as a patellar tibial free graft with attached bone blocks. A variation developed by Marshall and colleagues [90] in 1979 used pre-patellar fascia and the quadriceps tendon, plus the central one third of the patellar tendon. In 1982, Clancy and colleagues [91] published the results of an autogenous ACL reconstruction using the central one third of the patellar tendon by open arthrotomy. Classic biomechanical studies by Noyes and colleagues in 1984 [92,93] showed that 14 mm of the patellar tendon was biomechanically superior to other autogenous substitutes. In 1987, graft fixation in the femur was noted by Kurosaka and colleagues [94] to be superior to the 6.5 mm AO screw when a custom screw was inserted in an interference fashion. In 1993, Buss and colleagues [95] from the Hospital of Special Surgery reported that the arthroscopic-assisted ACL reconstruction using the central one third patellar tendon allograph, like the open technique, produced satisfactory results in a 42-month period. There were two distinct disadvantages using the femoral drill hole method of patellar tendon-bone free graft. When drilling the femoral hole, a sharp edged corner results that may produce a stress failure of the tendon as the knee is flexed to 90°. By smoothing the edge, this problem can be avoided. The second problem noted was the possibility of guillotining of the graft unless the intercondylar notch is debrided (notchplasty). Both techniques now are fundamental. By 1996, Arciero and colleagues [96] reported that the arthroscopically assisted ACL reconstruction had become the procedure of choice.

ACL reconstruction with bone-patellar tendon-bone versus two-strand hamstring autograft, as reported by Beynnon and colleagues [97] in 2005, noted that the bone-patellar tendon-bone reconstruction had anterior-posterior (AP) laxity value closer to normal when compared with the two-strand hamstring method. It appears that, after review of the literature and as noted by Spindler and colleagues' [98] review, the four-strand hamstring procedure proved to be essentially equal to the bone patellar tendon bone graft in measurement of laxity knee scoring, especially when employing an endo-button fixation of the hamstring sling on the femur and screw fixation on a spiked washer on the tibia. It should be added that Aglietti [99] in 1997 and Feller and Webster [100] in 2003 noted increased AP laxity in hamstring reconstruction when followed for 4 or more years. Debate continues as to the proper type of ACL reconstruction in a child or adolescent with open growth plates. The best plan is to procrastinate and reduce risk factors, if possible.

Shoulder arthroscopy has followed the development parallel to that of the knee. Burman [84] reported direct visualization of several joints, including 25 shoulders in cadavers from both anterior and posterior portals. In 1918 Takagi in Japan used a 7.3 mm cystoscope to visualize cadaver joints, and is given credit for inaugurating the field of arthroscopy [101,102]. Before arthroscopy, aging of the rotator cuff was studied to elucidate the causes of shoulder pain and disease. Studies noted chemical degradation of tendons, hypovascularity, and diminution of the polysaccharides in the collagen fibers caused by the forces of demand caused by use and aging. The central attachment of the superspinatus to the greater tuberosity of the humerus and the biceps tendon were the possible sources of pathology. With the arthroscope and MRI, external and internal impingement were recognized. The more common anterior dislocation and the less frequent traumatic posterior dislocation were demonstrated, along with corresponding labral pathology. Bankart [19,103] described a tear in the anterior inferior labrum. Labral tears with posterior dislocation often are referred to as a reversed Bankart. The long head of the biceps attaches to the superior labrum. The biceps tendon/labrum tear was first described by Andrews and colleagues [104]. Further attention was drawn to the superior labrum by Snyder and coworkers [105] in 1990, Smith and colleagues [106] in 1993, Monu and coworkers [107] in 1994, and Morgan and colleagues [108] in 1998, and the superior labrum anterior-posterior (SLAP) lesion became a legend in its time. Arthroscopic reattachment of the labrum with absorbable tacks soon followed, with favorable results.

Popularity of the usefulness of elbow arthroscopy tarried behind that of the shoulder. Yet, a salient circumstance occurred in 1974, when Dr. Indelicato and colleagues performed a medial collateral ligament reconstruction of the elbow using the palmaris longus tendon graft fashioned, doubled and passed through drill holes in the humerus and the ulna [109]. The ulnar nerve was freed up proximally and buried under flexor muscles distally. The recipient, a left-handed pitcher, went on to pitch successfully for 4 more years. The operation, with variations, bears his name, Tommy John.

The role of the team physician, as stated by Dr. O'Donoghue [110] in 1972, simply was "to prevent injury, to minimize temporary disability and prevent permanent disability. The final goal is complete recovery." Dr. O'Donoghue continues to define the well-run athletic program, which consists of the coach, who understands the proceedings, the trainer, the team physician, and the specialist, all of whom combine to form an effective unit. The position of the teacher to the team, player, and other physicians is emphasized by Dr. O'Donoghue, who is considered to be the father of modern sports medicine in the United States. His book, *Treatment of Injuries to Athletes*, was considered the Bible for sports medicine physicians. Early examinations of the player, conservative treatment, and prompt referral to a specialist when the situation demands are his basic concepts.

In an editorial in the *American Journal of Sports Medicine* in 1979 [111], Dr. Hughston summarized the essence of the spectrum of a team physician as being involved: involved by giving time, interest, and mental and physical effort. There is a need to establish rapport with the players, coaches, trainers, and the administration. Hughston mentions that a concerted effort is necessary to get to know the athletes, their personalities, motivation, and pain tolerance. The team physician must increase knowledge of the sport, its equipment, and its techniques. It is the obligation of the team physician to make certain that all personnel are trained, have arranged for emergencies (ambulance/emergency medical technician), and have routine medical supplies and equipment on the sidelines. An exit plan and the location of specific emergency. facilities for each type of injury are essential. There must be assurance of prior arrangement of hospital availability and hospital privileges. Dr. Hughston concludes with the hallmarks of a good team physician, which are availability, compassion, gentleness, and a true love of being helpful to those who show good sportsmanship [111].

In 1973, Wilson [112] reported on the effectiveness of the team physician being dependent upon the joint effort of the athletes, their parents, officials, coaches, athletic trainers, and the school administration. Rapport with each is important, but the primary concerns for the team physician are prevention of athletic injuries, treatment of the medical/surgical problem, and complete rehabilitation. The importance of pre-participation medical examination is stressed, along with conditioning. Wilson mentioned good coaching, adequate nutrition, and close supervision of practices to maintain hydration and to prevent heat problems. Dr. Wilson advocated salt tablets, Kool-Aid–flavored water (to add calories and palatability) and K-Lyte for potassium. He proposed the wearing of properly fitting gear and shoes, taping ankles only for basketball (unless previously injured), and renounced spearing, grabbing the face mask, and pulling. Should physician coverage for high school football games not be available and rapidly accessible at practice, the county medical society must search locally and in another community for assistance. Dr. Wilson concludes by quoting the first part of the first line of the Bill of Rights as developed by the Committee on the Medical Aspect of Sports of the American Medical Association [113]: "Participation in athletics is a privilege."

From the attributes, duties and obligations as depicted by Dr. O'Donoghue, Dr. Hughston, and Dr. Wilson, it is obvious that the nature of the future team physician is quite specific and operational within certain boundaries. The team physician must be a licensed MD or DO in good graces in the local community and state, must have a keen desire for service to and appreciation of athletes, must have completed a sports medicine fellowship with board certification or qualified for certification in a specialty (medical or surgical), must have extended experience with NCAA-monitored school athletic programs, and must have the personality, patience, and family support to establish a long-term relationship with the school, college, or professional team.

The future team physician needs to possess administrative capabilities to formulate an efficient sports medicine team that includes athletic trainers/physical therapists, coaches, administrative staff, parents, local doctors, and referral specialists. Continuing education, in-house research planning and participation, and teaching student athletic trainers, while fine tuning diagnostic skills, are extremely important. Availability, coverage of events, and office hours must be balanced with a pleasant, rewarding home life. The training experienced in residency and in fellowship can be enhanced, polished, and applied with gusto to produce a very rewarding and pleasurable sojourn. The Team Physician Consensus Statement published in the *American Journal of Sports Medicine*, prepared by an illustrious, multispecialty group, assembled in 2000 [114] to define the team physician, is an excellent reference for added details and completeness. An international flavor is presented in a 1994 article by Lynch and Carcasona [115] in the Football International Olympic Committee Handbook series. McBryde and Barfield [116] provide an excellent short summary of sports medicine in their 2006 *Southern Medical Journal* article.

In 2005, Dr. Steiner's group at Harvard published a study [117] that identified the clinical activities of the medical team physician who cares for intercollegiate athletic programs. Not chronicled were teaching sessions with coaches, athletic trainers, and athletes on injury prevention and nutritional topics. Although the team physician cares for a wide variety of problems, the visits to the health center office were predominately for musculoskeletal injuries such as contusions, sprains, and strains. Of the injuries that were significant, only 4% of the total required surgery. The ability to read radiographs, EKGs, and MRIs, plus the expertise to arrive at a working diagnosis, and plan and supervise rehabilitation are critical to success of the program. Of course, the physician planning a future as a medical team physician must be well versed in treating common entities such as respiratory (sinus and allergy) symptoms, skin eruptions, nutritional situations, headaches, and fatigue. To be able to diagnose both an acute abdomen and a torn ACL is a measure of sports medicine competency. Dr. Steiner believes that the specialty of internal medicine is more aptly suited for the position of medical team physician, basically because the boarded individual most likely will not need to obtain specialty assistance [117]. Thank goodness that this opinion was not adhered to when author Whiteside, a pediatrician, accepted the team physician's appointment at Pennsylvania State University, in University Park, in 1974.

Consider a typical family back in the early 1930s. The war to-end-all-wars was over. Beer was good and kept cool in a real ice box. The closest phone was next door. A stamp cost 3 cents. Dad had to join the union at work or get hurt. A son had just gotten out of house quarantine from scarlet fever. One neighbor kid had died of diphtheria and one kid at school had been crippled with polio. Evenings were spent listening to the one radio, enjoying life as Dad smoked his pipe while mom sewed peacefully. It was the Yankees against the Cubs in the 1932 World Series. The announcer described how Babe Ruth pointed to the fence and hit the next pitch for a homer. The family had high hopes for the future, but they did not have an inkling about what to expect. In fact, no thought was given. How could life be better?

Just imagine that family's bleak future without wide screen, high definition television, ubiquitous cell phones, color digital cameras, refrigerators/icemakers, air conditioning, and instant everything. No computer, bipod, DID, microwave, dishwasher, or pizza delivery. Vaccines and baby shots prevent contagious diseases. The iron lung of polio days is an antique. Most hospitals have sophisticated ECHO, radiograph, 16-slice CT, ultrasound, MRIs, and single-photon emission-computed topography isotope examinations. Doctors are now super specialists who take off weekends and send problems to the convenient emergency room. Movies and television sets entertain.

In so many ways, this present generation's typical family is similar to the folks in the early 1930s. Life is good. How could it be better overall? Kids drive their own cars to school. Dad and Mom are on a diet. No one ever dies of an illness. The conviction is that the future takes care of itself, magically, so why give it a thought? Just like the 1930s, nothing to be concerned about! What about bird flu, HIV, breast and prostate cancer, global warning, Iran as a nuclear power and social security running out of money, just to name a few?

The immediate future seems exceedingly positive, with the Human Genome Project having been successful in identifying the human genome. Genomic medicine will change health care by creating a fundamental understanding of the biology of many diseases, by creating pharmacogenomics, and to allow for genetic engineering and genetic stratification (marriage). Gene discovery speeds progeria and other congenital musculoskeletal research [118]. Genomic medicine is at the stage where knowledge of infection was 50 years ago. Men who have two copies of a mutated HPC1 gene have double the risk of developing prostate cancer [119]. Researchers have found a variant in a gene that is a genetic risk factor for developing Type II diabetes [120]. A form of doping as reported by the newspaper *The Australian*, [121] cites Oxford BioMedica (Oxford, England) for making Repoxygen, which allows the body to switch on a gene in response to low oxygen levels for the production of erythropoietin (EPO).

To reduce the source of musculotendinous pain and disability, research in the past has focused on developing new surgical techniques. Recently, attention has been directed toward understanding the biological milieu of the healing process of bone, cartilage, and tendon. In 1971, Urist and Strates [122] noted that certain proteins found at healing bone sites, when reintroduced, produced osteogenesis. These substances were named bone morphogenic proteins (BMP). Further research reported in 1994 by Storm and colleagues [123] and Chang and colleagues [124] and in 1997 by Wolfman and colleagues [125] identified three proteins as BMP 12, 13, and 14, each with different properties in animal experiments. BMP 12 was injected into rat partial Achilles ruptures, which when harvested revealed a definite increase in stiffness and strength.

In a laceration and repair of a long toe extensor tendon, BMP 12 was delivered to the area by an adenovirus gene. A 97% increase in tensile strength was reported. In a group of 50 rats, the Achilles tendon was transected and a 3 mm segment removed. BMP 13 was injected in 40 of the rats and when the tendons were tested, the BMP group revealed a 39% higher tensile strength. BMP 14 results were equally as significant in tendon healing and strengthening. Early research on BMP 7 has received approval from the Food and Drug Administration (FDA) for treatment of recalcitrant long-bone nonunion. BMP 2 is a standard component of the spine surgeon's armamentarium. Can rotator cuff investigation and use be too far away [122,123]?

Patients who have chronic myeloid leukemia have a genetic defect in which part of one gene (BCR) on chromosome 22 is fused with part of another gene (ABL) on chromosome 9. The fusion of the two into one chromosome (Philadelphia) causes overproduction of abnormal white blood cells. Medical inhibitors to stop fusion are in development. Verichip (Delray, Florida) is marketing implantable metal chips that are easily filled electronically with pertinent information about health, emergency numbers, and even wills. When scanned, an identification number is flashed on the computer that reveals the stored information. The company has marketed this chip successfully for animals since 1991. The American Medical Association (AMA) is reviewing the product and its use. The possibilities are endless. It is foreseeable that all newborn babies will be "chipped." This procedure allows parents (or a parole officer) to press the satellite remote pad and have the exact location of the person appear on the wrist color display, ready for audible communication. The parent or civil authority buys time on a satellite, which also allows for banking and grocery ordering.

Musculoskeletal operations will be robotic in nature. A technician will prepare the stereotaxic measurements and enter the data verbally into the computer. When dermal anesthesia has reached an effective level, the surgeon will place his disc into the robot, which will perform the surgery without an assistant. Family members follow the surgery by satellite view that is provided in the waiting rooms. Also, prosthetic engineering will enable spatial control of amputated limbs and facilitate ambulation without falling. Bioabsorbable plastic enhanced with bone morphogenic proteins will replace metal for fracture fixation [126].

Vaccines, in addition to the routine for prevention of childhood illnesses, will be developed to prevent addiction to alcohol, tobacco, drugs, a life of crime, and overeating. Stem cell research, which has been lagging, will produce evidence to decrease musculoskeletal abnormalities and viral infections. DNA investigation will identify telomere extender pharmaceuticals that will prevent cellular senescence, and as a consequence enhance longevity [127]. There will be the ability to biopsy a specimen, rescue the cellular precursors, grow specific tissue in large amounts with the use of certain growth factors, apply the modified tissue to a lattice, and then implant the sculptured product. Use for this methodology will be used when a stint is introduced into the left anterior descending coronary artery (LADA) and a biopsy taken. A newly fabricated LADA could replace the clogged artery as easily as replacing the muffler on a 1976 corvette. Because obesity will be controlled, bariactric (bypass) elective surgery will become obsolete. Wars, strife, and use of illegal performance enhancing drugs will continue unabated until He comes, but otherwise, no one can conceive what marvels the future holds.

References

[1] Available at: http://en.wikipedia.org/wiki/Herodicus. Accessed August 2, 2006.

[2] Athletic injuries: prevention, diagnosis, and treatment. Thorndike A. Philadelphia: Lea & Febinger; 1948. p. 15, 18, 22, 23, 46.

[3] Darling EA. The effects of training. A study of the Harvard University crews. Boston Medical and Surgical Journal 1899;141(9):205.

[4] Nichols EH, Richardson FL. Football injuries of the Harvard squad for three years under the revised rules. Boston Medical and Surgical Journal 1909;160(2):33.

[5] Nichols EH, Smith HB. The physical aspects of American football. Boston Medical and Surgical Journal 1906;154(1):1.

[6] Available at: http://www.theodoreroosevelt.org/kidscorner/football.htm. Accessed August 2, 2006.

[7] Available at: www.ncaa.org. Accessed August 2, 2006.

[8] Tipton CM. Sports medicine: a century of progress. J Nutr 1997;127:878s–85s.

[9] Available at: http://www.fims.org/default.asp?PageID=483889893. Accessed August 2, 2006.

[10] Herxheimer H. Grundriss der Sportmedizin fur Arzte und Studierende. Leipzig (Germany): George Thieme; 1933.

[11] Eggleton P, Eggleton GP. The inorganic phosphate and a labile form of organic phosphate in the gastrocnemius of the frog. Biochem Journal 1927;21:190.

[12] Fiske CH, Subbarow Y. The nature of the "inorganic phosphate" in voluntary muscle. Science 1927;65:401.

[13] Hill AV. Revolution of muscle physiology. Physiology Review 1932;1:56.

[14] Talbott JH, Michelson J. Heat cramps, a clinical and chemical study. J Clin Invest 1933;12(5):533.

[15] Dill DB, Talbott JH, Edwards HT. Studies in muscular activity. J Physiol 1930;69(3):293.

[16] Ladell WSS. Thermal sweating. British Medical Bulletin 1945;3:175.

[17] Edwards HT, Wood WB. A study of leucocytosis in exercise. Eur J Appl Physiol 1932; 6(1–2):73–83.

[18] Hill AC, Long CNH, Lupton H. Muscular exercise; lactic acid, and the supply and utilization of oxygen. Proceedings of the Royal Society B 1924;96:438.

[19] Edwards HT, Thorndike A Jr, Dill DB. The energy requirement in strenuous muscular exercise. N Engl J Med 1935;213(11):532.

[20] Bankart ASBL. The pathology and treatment of recurrent dislocation of the shoulder joint. Br J Surg 1938;26:23–9.

[21] Cyriax CY. Pathology and treatment of tennis elbow. J Bone Joint Surg Am 1936;18(4): 921–40.

[22] Simon NT. Semilunar cartilage and the football knee. New Orleans Med Surg J 1936;89: 287.

[23] Johnson RE, Brouha L, Darling RC. A test of physical fitness for strenuous exertion. Rev Can Biol 1942;1(5):491.

[24] Welch JE. Pioneering in health education and services at Amherst College. J Am Coll Health 1982;30:289–95.

[25] Hellebrandt FA, Karpovich PV. Fitness, fatigue, and recuperation: survey of methods used for improving the physical performance of man. War Med 1941;1:745–68.

[26] Quigley TB. Some observations on prevention and treatment of athletic injuries. Proceedings of the American College Health Association. Philadelphia, 1957.

[27] Schneider EC, Karpovich PV. Physiology of muscular activity. Philadelphia: WB Saunders; 1948.

[28] Cureton TK Jr. Physical fitness of champion athletes. Urbana (II): University of Illinois; 1951.

[29] Delorme T, Watkins A. Techniques of progressive resistance exercise. Arch Phys Med Rehabil 1948;29:263–73.

[30] Dutoit GT, Ensilin TB. Analysis of one hundred consecutive arthrotomies for traumatic internal derangement of the knee joint. J Bone Joint Surg Am 1945;27:412.

[31] Hey W. On internal derangement of the knee. In: Practical observations in surgery. London: Hansard; 1803. p. 332–41.

[32] Pendergrass EP, Lafferty JO. Roentgen study of ankle in severe sprains and dislocations. Radiology 1945;45:40.

[33] Bosworth BML. Acromioclavicular separation. Surgical forum. Bull Am Coll Surg 1947; 32:86.

[34] Bennett GE. Shoulder and elbow lesions distinctive of baseball players. Ann Surg 1947; 1276:107.

[35] Andrews JR, Hackel JG, Reinold MM, et al. Thrower's exostosis pathophysiology and management. Techniques in Shoulder and Elbow Surgery 2004;5(1):44–50.

[36] Keefer C. Antibiotic agents in clinical medicine. R I Med J 1947;30:579.

[37] Hughston JC. The role of the team physician. In: Baker CL Jr, editor. The Hughston Clinic sports medicine book. Philadelphia: Willliams & Wilkins; 1995. p. vii–ix, 3–4.

[38] Brav EA, Gulledge WH. Impressions concerning Putti-Platt reconstruction operation for recurrent shoulder dislocation. Surgery 1951;29:82–96.

[39] Helfet AJ. Coracoid transplantation for recurring dislocations of the shoulder. J Bone Joint Surg Br 1958;40:198.

[40] McLaughlin HL. Lesion of the musculotendinious cuff of the shoulder. Trauma. Philadelphia: WB Saunders Co.; 1959. p. 254.

[41] Quigley TB. Injuries of the hand, wrist, forearm and elbow sustained in college athletics. Instr Course Lect 1960;17:368.

[42] Thompson WAL, Glick IV, Silverstein DC. Buccal amylase new inflammatory agent. Clin Orthop Relat Res 1960;18:244.

[43] Schneider RC, Reifel E, Crisler HO, et al. Serious and fatal football injuries involving the head and spinal cord. JAMA 1961;177:362.

[44] Rose KD, Schneider PJ, Sullivan GF. A liquid pre-game diet for athletes. JAMA 1961;178: 30.

[45] Stenger JM, Lawson EA, Wright IM, et al. Mouthguards: protection against shock to head, neck and teeth. J Am Dent Assoc 1967;74(4):735–40.

[46] Available at: http://www.titleix.info/. Accessed August 2, 2006.

[47] Wels S. The Olympic spirit: 100 years of the games. Del Mar (CA): Tehabi Books; 1995.

[48] Ryan A. Medical services for the modern Olympic games. In: Ryan AJ, Allman FL, editors. Sports medicine. San Diego (CA): Academic Press; 1989. p. 3–21.

[49] Slocum D, Larson R. Pes anserinus transplantation. J Bone Joint Surg Am 1968;50: 226–42.

[50] Nicholas J. The five-one reconstruction for anteromedial instability of the knee: indications, technique, and the results in fifty-two patients. J Bone Joint Surg Am 1973;55:899–922.

[51] Hughston JC, Andrews JR, Cross MJ, et al. Classification of knee ligament instabilities. Part I. Medial compartment and cruciate ligaments. J Bone Joint Surg Am 1976;58: 159–72.

[52] Hughston JC, Andrews JR, Cross MJ, et al. Classification of knee ligament instabilities. Part II. The lateral compartment. J Bone Joint Surg Am 1976;58:173–9.

[53] Ellison A. Distal iliotibial band transfer for anterolateral rotatory instability of the knee. J Bone Joint Surg Am 1979;61:330–7.

[54] Andrews J, Sanders RA. A minireconstruction technique in treating anterolateral rotatory instability (ALRI). Clin Orthop 1983;172:93–6.

[55] Pringle JH. Avulsion of the sprine of the tibia. Ann Surg 1907;46:169.

[56] Jones R, Smith SA. On rupture of the crucial ligaments of the knee and on fractures of the spine of the tibia. Br J Surg 1913;1:70.

[57] Alwyn Smith S. The diagnosis and treatment of injuries to the crucial ligaments. Br J Surg 1918;6:176.

[58] Snook GA. The father of sports medicine. Am J Sports Med 1978;6(3):128–31.

[59] Bonnet A. Traité des maladies des articulations. vols. 1 and 2 with atlas Baillière; Paris: 1845.

[60] Noulis G. Entorse du genou. Thèse No 142. Faculté de Médecube de Oarus. Paris: Derenne; 1875. p. 1–53.

[61] Torg J, Conrad W, Kalen V. Clinical diagnosis of anterior cruciate ligament instability in the athlete. Am J Sports Med 1976;4:84–96.

[62] Mayo Robson AW. Ruptured crucial ligaments and their by operation. Am Surg 1903;37: 716.

[63] Hey Groves EW. The crucial ligaments of the knee joint: their function, rupture, and the operative treatment of the same. Br J Surg 1920;7:505.

[64] Galway H, MacIntosh DL. The lateral pivot shift: a symptom and sign of anterior cruciate ligament insufficiency. Clin Orthop 1980;147:45–50.

[65] Lange F. Über die Sehnenplastik. Verhandlungen der Deutschen Orthopaedic Gesellschaft 1903;2:10–2 [Dutch].

[66] Corner EM. The role of the crucial ligaments in haemarthrus and injuries to the knee. Lancet 1914;1:317.

[67] Ludloff K. Der operative Ersatz des vorderen Kreuzbandes am Knie. Zentralbl Chir 1927;54:3162–6 [German].

[68] Galeazzi R. La ricostituzione dei legamenti crociati del ginocchiuo. Atti e Memorie della Società Lombarda di Chirurgia 1934;XIII:302–317 [Italian].

[69] Jones K. Reconstruction of the anterior cruciate loigament using the central one-third of the patellar ligament. J Bone Joint Surg Am 1963;45:925–32.

[70] Bruckner H. Eine neue Methode zur Kreuzbandplastik. Chirgurgie 1966;37:413–4 [German].

[71] Milch H. Injuries to the crucial ligaments. Arch Surg 1935;30:805.

[72] Herzmark MHL. The evolution of the knee joint. J Bone Joint Surg Am 1938;20:77.

[73] Allman F. Sports medicine. New York: Academic Press; 1974.

[74] Fetto JF, Marshall JL. The natural history and diagnosis of anterior cruciate ligament insuffuency. Clin Orthop 1980;147:29.

[75] Palmer I. On the injuries to the ligaments of the knee joint. A clinical study. Acta Chir Scand 1938;81(Suppl 53):2–282.

[76] Smillie IS. Injuries of the knee joint. Baltimore (MD): Williams & Wilkins; 1948.

[77] Kleinberg S. The injection of oxygen into joints for diagnosis. Am J Surg 1921;35:256.

[78] Kleinberg S. Pulmonary embolism following oxygen injection of the knee. JAMA 1927;127:172.

[79] Quaintance PA. Pneumoroentgenography of the knee joint. J Bone Joint Surg Am 1938;20:353.

[80] Lindblom K. The arthrographic appearance of the ligaments of the knee. Acta Radiologica (Stockh) 1938;19:582–600.

[81] Bircher E. Die Arthroendoskopie. Zentralbl Chir 1921;48:1460 [German].

[82] Bircher E. Beitrag zur Pathologie (arthritis deformans) und Diagnose der Meniscus-Verletzungen (Arthro Endoscopie). Brun's Beitrage zur klinische Chirurgie 1922;127: 239 [German].

[83] Kreuscher PH. Semilunar cartilage disease: a plea for the early recognition by means of the arthroscope and the early treatment of this condition. Ill Med J 1925;47:290.

[84] Burman MS. Arthroscopy or the direct visualization of joints. An experimental cadaver study. J Bone Joint Surg Am 1931;13:669–95.

[85] Finkelstein H, Mayer L. The arthroscope: a new method of examining joints. J Bone Joint Surg Am 1931;13:583.

[86] Watanabe M, Takeda S, Ikeuchi H. Atlas of arthroscopy. Tokyo: Igakushoin; 1957.

[87] Jackson RW, Abe I. The role of arthroscopy in the management of disorders of the knee. An analysis of 200 consecutive examinations. J Bone Joint Surg Br 1972;54:310–22.

[88] O'Connor RL. Arthroscopy in the diagnosis and treatment of acute ligament injuries of the knee. J Bone Joint Surg Am 1974;56:333–7.

[89] Franke K. Clinical experience in 130 cruciate ligament reconstructions. Orthop Clin North Am 1976;7:191–3.

[90] Marshall JL, Warren RF, Wickiewicz TL, et al. The anterior cruciate ligament: a technique of repair and reconstruction. Clin Orthop 1979;143:97–106.

[91] Clancy WG Jr, Nelson DA, Reider B, et al. Anterior cruciate ligament reconstruction using one-third of the patellar ligament, augmented by extra-articular tendon transfers. J Bone Joint Surg Am 1982;64:352.

[92] Noyes FR, Butler DL, Grood ES, et al. Biomechanical analysis of human ligament grafts used in knee ligament repairs and reconstructions. J Bone Joint Surg Am 1984;66:344.

[93] Noyes FR, Keller CA, Grood ES, et al. Advances in the understanding of knee ligament injury, repair and rehabilitation. Med Sci Sports Exerc 1984;16:427.

[94] Kurosaka M, Yoshiya S, Andrish JA. A biomechanical comparison of different surgical techniques of graft fixation in anterior cruciate ligament reconstruction. Am J Sports Med 1987;15:225–9.

[95] Buss D, Warren R, Wickiewicz T, et al. Arthtoscopically assisted reconstruction of the anterior cruciate ligament with use of autogenous patellar ligament grafts: results after twenty-four to forty-two months. J Bone Joint Surg Am 1993;75:1346–55.

[96] Arciero RA, Scoville CR, Snyder RJ, et al. Single versus two-incision arthroscopic anterior cruciate ligament reconstruction. Arthroscopy 1996;12(4):462–9.

[97] Beynnon BD, Johnson RJ, Abate JA, et al. Treatment of anterior cruciate ligament injuries, part 1. Am J Sports Med 2005;33(10):1579–602.

[98] Spindler KP, Kuhn JE, Freedman KB, et al. Anterior cruciate ligament reconstruction autograft choice: bone-tendon-bone versus hamstring. Does it really matter? A systematic review. Am J Sports Med 2004;32(8):1986–95.

[99] Aglietti P, Buzzu R, Giron F, et al. Arthroscopic-assisted anterior cruciate ligament reconstruction with the central third patellar tendon. A 5-8 year follow-up. Knee Surg Sports Traumatol Arthrosc 1997;5(3):138–44.

[100] Feller JA, Webster KE. A randomized comparison of patellar tendon and hamstring tendon anterior cruciate ligament reconstruction. Am J Sports Med 2003;31(4):564–73.

[101] Takagi K. Practical experience using Takagi's arthroscope. Journal of the Japanese Orthopaedic Association 1933;8:132 [in Japanese].

[102] Takagi K. The arthroscope. Journal of the Japanese Orthopaedic Association 1939;14: 359–441 [in Japanese].

[103] Bankart ASB. Recurrent or habitual dislocation of the shoulder joint. British Journal of Medicine 1923;2:1132.

[104] Andrews JR, Carson WG Jr, McLeod WD. Glenoid labrum tears related to the long head of the biceps. Am J Sports Med 1985;13(5):337–41.

[105] Snyder SJ, Karzel RP, Del Pizzo W, et al. SLAP lesions of the shoulder. Arthroscopy 1990;6(4):274–9.

[106] Smith AM, McCauley TR, Jokl P. SLAP lesions of the glenoid labrum diagnosed with MR imaging. Skeletal Radiol 1993;22(7):507–10.

[107] Monu JU, Pope TL Jr, Chabon SJ, et al. MR diagnosis of superior labral anterior posterior (SLAP) injuries of the glenoid labrum: value of routine imaging without intraarticular injection of contrast material. AJR Am J Roentgenol 1994;163(6):1425–9.

[108] Morgan CD, Burkhart SS, Palmeri M, et al. Type II SLAP lesions: three subtypes and their relationships to superior instability and rotator cuff tears. Arthroscopy 1998;14(6): 553–65.

[109] Indelicato PA, Jobe FW, Kerlan RK, et al. Correctable elbow lesions in professional baseball players: a review of 25 cases. Am J Sports Med 1979;7(1):72–5.

[110] O'Donoghue DH. Treatment of injuries to athletes. Philadelphia: WB Saunders; 1972. p. 5.

[111] Hughston JC. Want to be in sports medicine? Get involved. Am J Sports Med 1979;7(2): 79–80.

[112] Wilson FC. The role of the physician in sports medicine. N C Med J 1973;34(1):38–43.

[113] Quigley TB. Some observations on prevention and treatment of athletic injuries. Presented at the Proceedings of the American College Health Associaton. Philadelphia, 1957.

[114] Team physician consensus statement. Am J Sports Med 2000;28(3):440–1.

[115] Lynch JM, Carcasona CB. The team physician. In: Ekblom B, editor. Football international Olympic committee handbook. Oxford (England): Blackwell Scientific Publications; 1994. p. 166–74.

[116] McBryde AM, Barfield B. Sports medicine: the last 100 years. South Med J 2006;99(7): 790.

[117] Steiner ME, Quigley B, Wang F, et al. Team physicians in college athletics. Am J Sports Med. 2005;33:1545–51.

[118] Kuehn BM. Gene discovery speeds progeria research. JAMA 2006;295:876–8.

[119] Casey G, Neville PJ, Plummer SJ, et al. RNASEL Arg462Gln variant is implicated in up to 13% of prostate cancer cases. Nat Genet 2002;32(4):581–3.

[120] Grant SF, Thorleifsson G, Reynisdottir I, et al. Variant of transcription factor 7-like 2 (TCF7L2) gene confers risk of type 2 diabetes. Nat Genet 2006;38(3):320–3.

[121] Available at: http://www.theaustralian.news.com.au/story/0,20867,18021974–2722,00.html. Accessed August 2, 2006.

[122] Urist MR, Strates BS. Bone morphogenetic protein. J Dent Res 1971;50(6):1392–406.

[123] Storm EE, Huynh TV, Copeland NG, et al. Limb alterations in brachypodism mice due to mutations in a new member of the TGF beta-superfamily. Nature 1994;14;368(6472): 639–43.

[124] Chang SC, Hoang B, Thomas JT, et al. Cartilage-derived morphogenetic proteins. New members of the transforming growth factor-beta superfamily predominantly expressed in long bones during human embryonic development. J Biol Chem. 1994;11;269(45): 28227–34.

[125] Wolfman NM, Hattersley G, Cox K, et al. Ectopic induction of tendon and ligament in rats by growth and differentiation factors 5, 6, and 7, members of the TGF-beta gene family. J Clin Invest 1997;100(2):321–30.

[126] Short PL. Building a business on biodegradability. Chemical & Engineering News 2006;84(28):12.

[127] Available at: http://www.geron.com/showpage.asp?code=prodta. Accessed September 18, 2006.

Clin Sports Med 26 (2007) 305–309

CLINICS IN SPORTS MEDICINE

EVIER
NDERS

INDEX

Note: Page numbers of article titles are in **boldface** type.

0278-5919/07/$ – see front matter
doi:10.1016/S0278-5919(07)00033-6

© 2007 Elsevier Inc. All rights reserved.
sportsmed.theclinics.com